Introduction to Pharmaceutical Calculations

Introduction to Pharmaceutical Calculations

Fourth edition

Judith A Rees BPharm, MSc, PhD
Senior Lecturer
School of Pharmacy
University of Keele, UK

Ian Smith BSc, MRPharmS, PGDip
Lecturer in Pharmacy Practice
School of Pharmacy
University of Keele, UK

Jennie Watson BSc (Hons), PGDip, PGCert (LTHE)
Boots Teacher Practitioner
University of Central Lancashire, UK

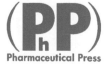

Pharmaceutical Press

Published by Pharmaceutical Press

66-68 East Smithfield, London E1W 1AW, UK

© Pharmaceutical Press 2015

(**PP**) is a trade mark of Pharmaceutical Press
Pharmaceutical Press is the publishing division of the Royal Pharmaceutical Society of Great Britain

First edition published 2001
Second edition published 2005
Third edition 2011
Fourth edition 2015
Fourth edition reprinted 2016, 2017, 2018, 2019, 2020, 2021, 2024

Typeset by Laserwords Private Limited, Chennai, India
Printed in Great Britain by TJ Books Limited, Padstow, Cornwall
Videos commissioned by Pharmaceutical Press
Videos produced by Designers Collective

ISBN 978 0 85711 168 5 (print)
ISBN 978 0 85711 243 9 (ePDF)
ISBN 978 0 85711 244 6 (epub)
ISBN 978 0 85711 245 3 (Mobi)

A catalogue record for this book is available from the British Library.

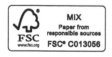

MIX
Paper from
responsible sources
FSC
www.fsc.org   FSC® C013056

Dedication

'No man dies until he is forgotten'

We would like to dedicate this book to the memory of Brian Smith who died suddenly on 11 March 2000. Without his ideas related to the teaching and learning of mathematics this book would not and could not have happened. He has been greatly missed by his wife and children, his grandchildren and everyone who knew him.

Contents

Preface

The first edition of this book was written because it became apparent, to us and others, that many pharmacy undergraduate students were experiencing difficulties when performing pharmaceutical calculations. Since that time it would appear that students still face the same difficulties with calculations, despite changes to the curriculum in UK schools. The importance of being able to confidently and accurately perform pharmaceutical calculations has been further emphasised by the General Pharmaceutical Council. Their Registration Assessment includes a section on calculations, which must be passed in its own right in order to qualify as a pharmacist. This requirement means that, even after graduation, preregistration trainees must hone their skills in pharmaceutical calculations. This book is produced in the hope that it will help and support pharmacy students, preregistration trainees, pharmacists, technicians and other healthcare professionals to carry out pharmaceutical calculations in a reliable and skilful manner and so avoid errors that may lead to potential patient harm.

The approach we have taken throughout the book is to use one method based on proportional sets to solve the various types of pharmaceutical calculation likely to be encountered in everyday pharmacy practice. This approach involves the initial organisation of given and required data from a question into proportional sets. This process allows the individual to sort out what is required by the question. Once the proportional set has been established, the application of simple algebra will then enable the determination of the unknown value. Ideally, the calculated value should be placed back into the proportional set, when it will become apparent whether or not the result is about the 'right' size: an important accuracy check if errors are to be avoided.

Although we realise that there may be several arithmetical ways to solve pharmaceutical calculations, by using one method for all different types of calculations we hope to reduce apprehensions/concerns about calculations and provide a consistent method of tackling all pharmaceutical calculations. In addition, the proportional sets approach enables a simple checking procedure to be put into place.

In the new edition we have updated material and added an initial explanatory chapter. We have also expanded the information about calculation of doses, with one chapter for adults and one chapter for children. Within each chapter we have also tried to set the scene more for the reader by relating the type of calculation to practice.

The layout of the book is, first, to introduce the reader to the proportional sets approach to solving calculations and, second, to explain the system of units used in pharmacy and the conversion between units. Third, the main part of the book applies the proportional sets approach and the system of units to pharmaceutical examples in the following topics:

- concentrations
- simple, serial and multiple dilution of solids and liquids
- reduction and enlargement of formulae for pharmaceutical products
- calculations involving concentrated waters and flavours
- doses and dosage regimens in children and adults
- displacement volumes and values
- density
- molecular weight
- parenteral solutions
- isotonicity
- accuracy of measurement including limits on pharmaceutical substances and preparations
- calculations involving information retrieval.

Fourth, the final part of the book is a series of appendices on long division, multiplication and how to deal with fractions, and general information.

We have also welcomed a new member to our team in Jennie Watson who is an experienced pharmacist and teacher practitioner.

Throughout the book up-to-date worked examples are clearly laid out and practice calculations with answers are provided at the end of each chapter. The companion text *Pharmaceutical Calculations Workbook* is also available (see www.pharmpress.com for more details).

The design of the book presents material in a clear way, so that readers can use the whole book as a learning resource or can use sections of the book for reference or to check understanding. We hope that this book will enable those involved in pharmaceutical calculations to perform them accurately and with confidence.

Judith Rees, Ian Smith and Jennie Watson
Manchester, 2015

Videos

In collaboration with the authors, Pharmaceutical Press have produced a series of eight short videos covering:

Simple dilution

Proportional sets

Conversion of units

Representations of concentrations

Mixing two concentrations without a final volume

Displacement values

Parenteral doses

Moles

Where you see this symbol in the book you are in a section where there is an accompanying video.

Visit www.pharmpress.com/calculationsvideos and enter the code: **calculations** to view the videos.

Acknowledgement

We wish to express our indebtedness to the late Richard Skemp on whose work the proportional sets approach to rational numbers used in this book is based.

About the authors

Judith A Rees studied pharmacy in Bradford before completing a PhD in Manchester. Until recently she was a senior lecturer in the School of Pharmacy and Pharmaceutical Sciences at the University of Manchester. She is currently senior lecturer in the School of Pharmacy at Keele University.

Ian Smith studied pharmacy in Manchester. He is now a lecturer in Pharmacy Practice at Keele University. Prior to that he was a Boots Teacher Practitioner.

Jennie Watson studied pharmacy in Brighton. She carried out a variety of roles for Boots before becoming their Teacher Practitioner at the University of Central Lancashire.

1

Introduction

Pharmacists provide the final safety check before medicines reach the patient. During your time at university as a pharmacy student and during your preregistration year, you will develop many skills to help you minimise the risk of the medicine you supply harming a patient. The ability to accurately carry out pharmaceutical calculations is one of these skills.

As a student, it is easy to become engrossed in the mathematical side of the calculation and forget that the purpose of the calculation is to ensure the patient receives the correct product at the appropriate strength with appropriate dosing instructions. Throughout this book we have therefore tried to relate the chapters back to the circumstances in practice in which you may need to use the particular type of calculation.

We have also observed students over many years trying to overcomplicate pharmaceutical calculations when they carry them out. We understand that while you are a student, complicated mathematics are required in other parts of your course, for example in statistics and pharmaceutics. The mathematics needed for pharmaceutical calculations is of a much more basic level and primarily requires you to be able to add, subtract, multiply and divide. This is one of the reasons you are encouraged or expected to be able to carry out these calculations without the aid of a calculator. The General Pharmaceutical Council supports this recommendation. It may have been a long time since you attempted mathematical problems without a calculator and you may have forgotten some of the methods, in particular, when asked to multiply or divide a number. As a reminder we have produced Appendix 3, which reminds you how to carry out both multiplication and long division.

We understand that for some of you, calculations are never going to be a topic of choice. If you feel like this, you need to consider whether you could think about numbers on a regular basis. Being comfortable with basic numeracy is a skill that can, like many skills, be developed through practice. Like any new skill, try to develop it slowly but regularly:

- add up your bill in a café while standing in the queue;
- if you carry out some exercise, keep working out how far you are towards your target as a percentage, decimal or fraction of that target;
- keep a check on how much money you have got left in your bank account by keeping a running balance in your head.

You will need to do these activities without the aid of a calculator in order to get any benefit.

The other reason you are required to work without a calculator is to encourage you to sense-check your calculation and final answer. We encourage you to do this because it will help you think about the calculation in real rather than abstract terms. Consider the following:

You are asked to express the strength of salbutamol syrup 2 mg/5 mL as a percentage.

Percentage calculations require you to work only in grams and millilitres. If you didn't remember this rule, it would be very easy to tap numbers into a calculator and decide that the answer is a percentage strength of 40%, i.e.

$$(2 \div 5) \times 100\% = 40\%$$

If you then 'sense-checked' this answer you would realise that 40% is unlikely to be the answer because 40% solutions are rarely possible due to the solubility of the solute in the solvent.

Alternatively consider the figure below:

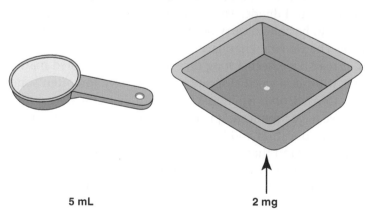

5 mL   2 mg

If you placed the 2 mg on the 5 mL spoon it would not fill nearly half the spoon so 40% must be the wrong answer.

Similarly if your answer tells you that you can dissolve 300 g in 100 mL, then thinking sensibly this answer is also highly likely to be incorrect.

Before we go any further, it is also important to think about units of weight and volume. We cover some of the detail of using units in Chapter 3 but there are some important basic pieces of information you need to be very comfortable with before you start.

Firstly the size order of the units:

Weight:

kg > g > mg > microgram

All by a factor of 1000 between each unit.

Volume:

L > mL

Again by a factor of 1000.

It is also very helpful to be able to relate abstract weights and volumes to real objects so here are some examples:

1 grain of salt weighs about 2 mg

1 small paperclip weighs about 1 gram

20 sugar cubes weigh about 100 grams

1 average melon or pineapple weighs about 1 kg

1 teaspoon holds just under 5 mL of water

A standard can of fizzy drink contains 330 mL

But before we start the real calculations, take time to remind yourself that numbers work in a logical way – they follow simple patterns and orders – and if you also work in a straightforward and logical way, you will be capable of successfully and accurately carrying out pharmaceutical calculations.

2

Rational numbers

Learning objectives

By the end of this chapter you will be able to:

- convert a number from a decimal to a fraction or a percentage
- identify proportional sets
- express fractions in their lowest terms
- set up a proportional set and find the missing value using three different methods

Most students will already have at least a basic knowledge of arithmetic and algebra, so the aim of this chapter is to provide a reinforcement of the particular mathematical concepts that are necessary in order to carry out the calculations required in pharmacy. School mathematics courses tend to treat the basic tools of fractions, decimals and percentages as quite separate topics. In this book an attempt is made to provide a more unified and hopefully a more interesting approach.

Proportional sets of numbers

Consider the following sets of data:

A drug is in solution at a concentration of 75 mg to 5 mL:

weight of drug (mg)	15	30	45	60	75	90...
volume of solution (mL)	1	2	3	4	5	6...

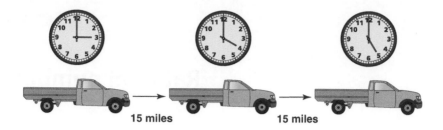

A heavy vehicle travels at a steady speed of 15 miles per hour:

distance travelled (miles)   15   30   45   60   75   90...

time taken (hours)   1   2   3   4   5   6...

In these two sets of data we see that the numbers are the same. The same arrangement of numbers serves as an image for two quite different practical situations.

Let us extract the two sets of numbers:

set A   15   30   45   60   75   90...

set B   1   2   3   4   5   6...

We see that there is a relationship between the two sets: each number in set A is 15 times the corresponding number in set B.

When one set of numbers is obtained by multiplying each number of the other set by a fixed number, the two sets are said to be *proportional*. Thus we can say that set A is proportional to set B.

Now consider the next two sets of numbers:

3   5   9...

12   20   36...

In this example each lower number is obtained by multiplying the corresponding upper number by 4. Again the two sets are proportional.

Now consider the next two sets of numbers:

3   8   13   18...

1   2   3   4...

There is no fixed number by which the lower set of values can be multiplied in order to arrive at corresponding values of the upper set or vice versa. The two sets are not proportional to each other.

Examples 2.1–2.5

In each of the following questions decide whether or not the pairs of sets are proportional.

2.1   6   10   14
               3   5   7

Proportional. Each value of the upper set is twice the corresponding value of the lower set.

2.2   5   7   9
               40   56   72

Proportional. Each value of the lower set is eight times the corresponding value of the upper set.

2.3   2   4   8
               1   2   3

Not proportional.

2.4   5   7   9
               15   17   19

Not proportional.

2.5   16   17   21
               80   85   105

Proportional. Each value of the lower set is five times the corresponding value of the upper set.

Ratios

Proportional sets can be used to explain the term 'ratio'.
    For the proportional sets:

        9   21   30   36...
        3   7   10   12...

each number in the upper set is three times the corresponding number in the lower set. Each of the corresponding pairs of numbers is said to be in the ratio three to one.

For the next pair of proportional sets:

2   5   7...

10   25   35...

one to five is the ratio of the corresponding pairs. The ratio one to five can also be expressed as 1: 5.

Numbers that represent ratios are called *rational numbers*. Fractions, decimals and percentages are three kinds of numerals that can be used to represent rational numbers. We will examine the relationships between these three different notations.

Fractions

The ratio 4 to 1 is represented by the fraction $\frac{4}{1}$, which is equivalent to the natural number 4. (The *natural numbers* are the counting numbers $1, 2, 3 \ldots$)

The ratio 1 to 5 is represented by the fraction $\frac{1}{5}$. The number on top of a fraction is called the numerator and the bottom number is the denominator:

$$\text{fraction} = \frac{\text{numerator}}{\text{denominator}}$$

Consider the proportional sets:

1   2   3   4...

5   10   15   20...

We can see that ratio 1 to 5 = ratio 2 to 10 = ratio 3 to 15 and so on. As each ratio can be represented by a fraction, we can write down as many different names as we wish for any given fraction:

$$\frac{1}{5} = \frac{2}{10} = \frac{3}{15} = \frac{4}{20} = \frac{5}{25} \text{ and so on.}$$

To obtain other names for a given fraction we multiply (or divide) both numerator and denominator by the same number.

Example 2.6

Find the numerator of the fraction that is equal to $\frac{1}{7}$ but has denominator 21.

Let the numerator be x:

$$\frac{1}{7} = \frac{x}{21}$$

Denominator 7 has been multiplied by 3 to get new denominator 21, so numerator 1 must be multiplied by 3 to get x, therefore $x = 3$.
   The numerator is 3.

Example 2.7

Find the numerator of the fraction that is equal to $\frac{16}{24}$ but has denominator 3.

Let the numerator be y:

$$\frac{y}{3} = \frac{16}{24}$$

Denominator 24 has been divided by 8 to get new denominator 3, so numerator 16 must be divided by 8 to get y, therefore $y = 2$.
   The numerator is 2.

Example 2.8

Find the denominator of the fraction that is equal to $\frac{80}{180}$, but has numerator 16.

Let the denominator be x:

$$\frac{16}{x} = \frac{80}{180}$$

Numerator 80 has been divided by 5 to get 16, so x is 180 divided by 5, therefore $x = 36$.
   The denominator is 36.

Fractions expressed in their lowest terms

As there are many names for the same fraction, the one we tend to use to represent the fraction is the one for which there is no whole number that will divide exactly into both the numerator and the denominator. The fraction is then said to be expressed in its lowest terms.

Example 2.9

Express $\frac{35}{45}$ in its lowest terms.

Both 35 and 45 can be divided by 5. We divide numerator and denominator by 5 to get $\frac{7}{9}$.

Example 2.10

Express $\frac{60}{405}$ in its lowest terms.

We can see that 60 and 405 will divide by 5, so:

$$\frac{60}{405} = \frac{12}{81}$$

Now 12 and 81 will divide by 3, so:

$$\frac{60}{405} = \frac{12}{81} = \frac{4}{27}$$

Multiplication of a fraction by a whole number

We have seen that, if both the numerator and the denominator of a fraction are multiplied by the same number, the resulting fraction is equal to the first one and is just another name for it. To multiply a fraction by a whole number (an *integer*) we multiply only the numerator by the integer. Thus:

$$\frac{4}{7} \text{ multiplied by 3 becomes } \frac{12}{7}$$

$$\frac{5}{9} \text{ multiplied by 7 becomes } \frac{35}{9}$$

When $\frac{6}{7}$ is multiplied by 8 the result is $\frac{48}{7}$, which can be written as $\frac{42}{7} + \frac{6}{7} = 6\frac{6}{7}$.

Decimals

In the number 127, the 1 represents one hundred, the 2 represents two tens and the 7 represents seven units. The value of each digit is therefore dependent on its position in the number. This system of 'place values' is extended for the representation of decimals by introducing a decimal point after the unit value.

Units	.	Tenths	Hundredths	Thousandths	Ten-thousandths
0	.	2	3		
0	.	5	2	7	

The number 0.23 is a rational number. The 2 is in the tenths column and the 3 is in the hundredths column. Two tenths and three hundredths make twenty-three hundredths, so 0.23 is another name for the fraction $\frac{23}{100}$.

The number 0.527 has a 7 in the thousandths column so it is another name for the fraction $\frac{527}{1000}$.

For the reverse process, i.e. to express a fraction in decimal form, the numerator is simply divided by the denominator:

$$\frac{24}{64} = 24 \text{ divided by } 64 = 0.375.$$

Note that $\frac{2}{5}$, $\frac{4}{10}$ and $\frac{6}{15}$ are different names for the same fraction. Changing each fraction to a decimal:

2 divided by 5 = 4 divided by 10 = 6 divided by 15 = 0.4

Thus one decimal may be represented by many fractions.

Example 2.11

Convert 0.3 to a fraction.

The 3 is in the tenths column so $0.3 = \frac{3}{10}$.

Example 2.12

Convert 0.35 to a fraction.

The 5 is in the hundredths column so $0.35 = \frac{35}{100} = \frac{7}{20}$.

Example 2.13

Convert the fraction $\frac{3}{5}$ to a decimal.

3 divided by 5 gives 0.6 or:

$$\frac{3}{5} = \frac{6}{10} = 0.6$$

Example 2.14

Convert the fraction $\frac{7}{8}$ to a decimal.

7 divided by 8 gives 0.875.

Percentages

5 per cent means 5 per hundred, so 5% represents the same rational number as the fraction

$$\frac{5}{100} = \frac{5}{5 \times 20} = \frac{1}{20}$$

Similarly, 31% is the same as $\frac{31}{100}$.

    To change a fraction to a percentage, we can change the fraction to a decimal and then examine the decimal to see how many units there are in the hundredths column. The number of hundredths gives the percentage. For example, let us convert the fraction $\frac{1}{20}$ to a percentage. First divide 1 by 20 to get the decimal 0.05. There is a 5 in the hundredths column. Five hundredths is equal to 5%.

Similarly, the fraction $\frac{3}{40} = 3$ divided by $40 = 0.075$. There is a 7 in the hundredths column, so there are 7.5 hundredths, which is 7.5%.

Example 2.15

Express 0.76 as a percentage.

There is a 6 in the hundredths column:

$0.76 = 76$ hundredths $= 76\%$

Example 2.16

Express 0.769 as a percentage.

There is a 6 in the hundredths column:

$0.769 = 76.9$ hundredths $= 76.9\%$

Example 2.17

Express 20% as a fraction in its lowest terms.

$$20\% = \frac{20}{100} = \frac{1}{5}$$

Example 2.18

Express 0.2% as a fraction in its lowest terms.

$$0.2\% = \frac{0.2}{100} = \frac{2}{1000} = \frac{1}{500}$$

Example 2.19

Express $\frac{7}{10}$ as a percentage.

$$\frac{7}{10} = 0.70 = 70\%$$

Example 2.20

Express $\frac{3}{8}$ as a percentage.

$$\frac{3}{8} = 0.375 = 37.5\%$$

Finding a missing value from two proportional sets

Most of the calculations encountered in dispensing are dependent on being able to find missing values from sets of proportional numbers and we are now almost ready to tackle the method for doing this. We have looked at the different forms of rational numbers such as fractions, decimals and percentages that may be required in carrying out the tasks.

We need one more piece of work before we can proceed. Consider the following two proportional sets:

set A p q

set B r s

Let us take the sets formed by the values in the vertical columns and call them set C and set D. Thus we have:

set C p r

set D q s

As set A is proportional to set B, then we see that the ratio of p to r is equal to the ratio of q to s and this can be expressed as:

$$\frac{p}{r} = \frac{q}{s}$$

Multiplying both sides of the equation by rs gives:

$$ps = rq$$

Dividing both sides of this equation by qs gives:

$$\frac{p}{q} = \frac{r}{s}$$

This means that set C is proportional to set D.

Let us now re-state this important result:

	set C	set D
set A	p	q
set B	r	s

If set A is proportional to set B, then set C is proportional to set D.

Let us check the result with a specific example:

set A	2	10
set B	4	20

Each value of set B is twice the corresponding value of set A, so set A is proportional to set B.

Interchanging the horizontal and vertical columns:

set C	2	4
set D	10	20

Each value of set D is five times the corresponding value of set C, so set C is proportional to set D.

In finding missing numbers from proportional sets we will consider three methods and denote them method A, method B and method C. Method A is the general method, which can be used in all cases; methods B and C are applicable only to a limited number of cases, but in such cases they will provide a simpler approach.

Example 2.21

For the proportional sets:

7	y	9	10...
21	24	27	30...

find the missing value y.

Method A

We set up an equation using the value y and its corresponding value 24 along with any other corresponding pair. Corresponding pairs of values are in the same ratio so:

$$\frac{y}{24} = \frac{9}{27}$$

The value of the variable y will remain unchanged if both sides of this equation are multiplied by a constant. We multiply both sides of the equation by 24 to get rid of the fraction involving y:

$$24 \times \frac{y}{24} = 24 \times \frac{9}{27}$$

Multiplying the fractions by the whole numbers (see p. 10):

$$\frac{24y}{24} = \frac{216}{27}$$

This simplifies to give $y = 8$.

Note: this is the general method, which can be applied to any pair of proportional sets.
    This example also lends itself to solution by method B.

$\rightarrow$

Method B

In this method we 'spot' the relationship between the proportional sets. Each value of the lower set is three times the corresponding value of the upper set, so y times $3 = 24$, therefore $y = 8$.

Method B is the easier method to apply in the limited number of cases in which it is applicable.

Example 2.22

For the proportional sets:

> x 14
>
> 25 50

find the missing number x.

If we attempt to use method B, we find that there is no obvious number that 50 can be divided by to get 14, but we are able to apply method C.

Method C

From the result on p. 15, the two vertical sets of numbers are proportional. The ratio of 50 to 25 is 2, so the ratio of 14 to x is also 2.

14 is divided by 2 to give $x = 7$. Again we are able to 'spot' the answer.

Method A

Corresponding pairs of values are in the same ratio so:

$$\frac{x}{25} = \frac{14}{50}$$

The value of the variable x will remain unchanged if both sides of this equation are multiplied by a constant. We multiply both sides of the

(*continued*)

equation by 25 to get rid of the fraction involving x:

$$25 \times \frac{x}{25} = 25 \times \frac{14}{50}$$

$$\frac{25x}{25} = \frac{350}{50}$$

This simplifies to give $x = 7$

Example 2.23

For the proportional sets:

3	x
5	*8*

find the missing value x.

Method A is the more appropriate method this time. Corresponding pairs are in the same ratio, so

$$\frac{x}{8} = \frac{3}{5}$$

Multiplying both sides of the equation by 8:

$$8 \times \frac{x}{8} = 8 \times \frac{3}{5}$$

$$x = \frac{24}{5}$$

The missing value is four and four-fifths $= 4.8$.

Note: if this example is compared with Example 2.22, method A, we can see that this time a step has been missed out. Now that we understand what is happening in solving the algebraic fractional equation, we can probably miss out yet another step and go directly from:

$$\frac{x}{8} = \frac{3}{5}$$

$\rightarrow$

to:

$$x = \frac{24}{5}$$

We use this method in Example 2.24.

Example 2.24

For the pair of proportional sets:

z   9

6   15

find the missing value z.

Using method A, corresponding pairs of values are in the same ratio, so:

$$\frac{z}{6} = \frac{9}{15}$$

$$z = \frac{54}{15}$$

$$z = 3.6$$

Example 2.25

For the proportional sets:

37   52

7   z

find the missing number z.

Using method A, corresponding pairs of values are in the same ratio, so we could write:

$$\frac{37}{7} = \frac{52}{z}$$

(*continued*)

It would, however, make the fractional equation easier to solve if we were to write down the equivalent equation:

$$\frac{z}{52} = \frac{7}{37}$$

Then:

$$z = \frac{364}{37}$$

$$z = 9.837837\ldots$$

Correcting to three significant figures gives $z = 9.84$. See Chapter 12.

Example 2.26

Consider three sets each proportional to each other:

x	20
y	50
30	150

Find x and y.

Solving using method A we can write:

$$\frac{x}{30} = \frac{20}{150} \quad \text{and} \quad \frac{y}{30} = \frac{50}{150}$$

giving:

$$x = \frac{600}{150} = 4 \quad \text{and} \quad y = \frac{1500}{150} = 10$$

The fact that the vertical columns form two proportional sets could be used to give:

$$\frac{x}{20} = \frac{30}{150} \quad \text{and} \quad \frac{y}{50} = \frac{30}{150}$$

leading to the same values of x and y.

$\rightarrow$

The best approach in this case would be the use of the 'spotting' method C. The ratio of 150 to 30 is 5, so y is 50 divided by $5 = 10$ and x is 20 divided by $5 = 4$.

Example 2.27

Find the values of a and b in the following proportional sets:

a	25	110
12	b	22

The best approach is by the 'spotting' method B. The ratio of 110 to 22 is 5, so a is 5 times $12 = 60$ and b is 25 divided by $5 = 5$.

Example 2.28

Find the value of p in the two proportional sets:

36	9
22	P

The best approach is by the 'spotting' method C. The ratio of 36 to 9 is 4, so 22 is divided by 4 to give $p = 5.5$.

Example 2.29

Find the values of x and y in the three proportional sets:

24	6
x	15
64	Y

The best approach is by the 'spotting' method C. The ratio of 24 to 6 is 4, so x is 15 times $4 = 60$ and y is 64 divided by $4 = 16$.

Example 2.30

Find the values of y and z in the two proportional sets:

y   18   21

9   z   63

The best approach is by the 'spotting' method B. The ratio of 63 to 21 is 3, so y is 9 divided by 3 = 3 and z is 18 times 3 = 54.

Note: from this point we will refer to methods B and C as the 'spotting' methods and to method A as the general method.

Setting up proportional sets for practical situations

We can now calculate missing values from two proportional sets of numbers, so let us deal with the setting up of two proportional sets in solving practical examples.

For the purposes of this general introduction, let us give the two proportional sets the titles set A and set B. Each of the numbers used in set A must be in the same units and the units should be stated after the title. The same situation must apply for numbers in set B.

We first need to identify the number that needs to be found and represent it by a letter. Then three known values need to be identified. One of them must be the value of the second set that corresponds to the required unknown value of the first set. The other two will be any known pair of values (one from each set) that correspond.

General situation:

set A (units for set A)   unknown value   known value

set B (units for set B)   known value   known value

Thus, for a particular situation, the form could be:

sodium chloride (mg) x 450

water (mL)   12.5   50

Let us set up the proportional sets from the following example:

A suspension contains 120 mg of paracetamol in each 5 mL. Find the volume of suspension that contains 300 mg of paracetamol.

We said earlier: 'We first need to identify the number that needs to be found and represent it by a letter. Then three known values need to be identified. One of them must be the value of the second set that corresponds to the required unknown value of the first set. The other two will be any known pair of values (one from each set) that correspond.'

Applying this to the example: Let the volume of suspension required (mL) be x. The amount of paracetamol that corresponds to this (in mg) is 300. The known pair of corresponding values is made up of 5 mL and 120 mg.

Setting up the proportional sets:

| volume of suspension (mL) | x | 5 |
| amount of paracetamol (mg) | 300 | 120 |

We can now go on to solve for x.

Example 2.31

The recommended dose of phenytoin for a patient is 840 mg. An injection contains 50 mg/mL. What volume of injection is needed for the recommended dose?

Let the required volume of injection (mL) be y. The corresponding known value is 840 mg and the known corresponding pair is made up of 1 mL and 50 mg. Setting up the proportional sets:

| amount of phenytoin (mg) | 840 | 50 |
| volume of injection (mL) | y | 1 |

We can then go on to solve for y.

Example 2.32

1 L of aqueous solution contains 250 mL of syrup. How much syrup will be contained in 25 L of the solution?

Let the required amount of syrup in millilitres be x. Setting up proportional sets:

volume of syrup (mL)	250	x
volume of solution (L)	1	25

We can then go on to solve for x.

Example 2.33

25 g of ointment contains 5 g of calamine. How much calamine will be contained in 60 g of ointment?

Let the required mass of calamine in grams be y. Setting up proportional sets:

mass of calamine (g)	5	y
mass of ointment (g)	25	60

We can then go on to solve for y.

Note: when the unknown value has been calculated it should be entered in the proportional sets table in place of the letter representing it and the user should then examine the table to check that the size of the calculated value seems to agree with corresponding values.

Proportional sets that become trivial

Consider the following example:

Calculate the number of tablets required for 7 days if 12 tablets are used each day.

The reader will be able to give the number as 84, but note that the problem involves proportion and could be tackled as follows.

Let the required number of tablets be x. Setting up proportional sets:

number of tablets   12 x

number of days   1   7

We can 'spot' that 1 is multiplied by 12 to give 12, so 7 is multiplied by 12 to give $x = 84$. The number of tablets required is 84.

There is no virtue in going to the trouble of writing out proportional sets in cases such as this one, but it is useful to know that we are dealing with proportion.

Now consider the following example:

Find the volume of solution that contains 50 mg of a drug and has a concentration of 4 mg in 1 mL.

Many readers will be able to give the volume as 12.5 mL, but this time some readers would probably welcome the help they would gain by writing down proportional sets.

Let the required volume of solution be y mL:

amount of drug (mg)   4   50

volume of solution (mL)   1 y

We can 'spot' that 4 is divided by 4 to give 1, so 50 is divided by 4 to give y:

$$y = \frac{50}{4} = 12.5$$

The volume of solution is 12.5 mL.

In tackling questions that involve a lot of information, it may be worth writing down proportional sets, including some that turn out to be rather trivial, in order to organise the information. The path to a solution will then probably become more obvious.

Proportional sets

Practice calculations

Answers are given at the end of the chapter.

In questions 1 to 6 decide whether or not the pairs of sets are proportional.

Q1   6   8   10...

   3   5   7...

Q2   5   7   9...

   20   28   36...

Q3   2   3   4...

   5   6   7...

Q4   2   4   6...

   5   10   15...

Q5   25   35...

   5   7...

Q6   2   4   6...

   3   6   9...

Q7   Find the fraction that is equal to $\frac{7}{8}$ but has denominator 72.

Q8   Find the fraction that is equal to $\frac{4}{7}$ but has numerator 28.

Q9   Find the fraction that is equal to $\frac{2}{9}$ but has denominator 117.

Q10   Express $\frac{12}{20}$ in its lowest terms.

Q11   Express $\frac{3}{15}$ in its lowest terms.

Q12   Express $\frac{42}{54}$ in its lowest terms.

Q13   Express $\frac{78}{130}$ in its lowest terms.

Q14   Express $\frac{120}{42}$ in its lowest terms.

Q15   Multiply $\frac{3}{13}$ by 5.

Q16   Multiply $\frac{3}{17}$ by 4.

Q17 Multiply $\frac{5}{9}$ by 7.

Q18 Convert 0.8 to a fraction in its lowest terms.

Q19 Convert 0.87 to a fraction in its lowest terms.

Q20 Convert 0.875 to a fraction in its lowest terms.

Q21 Convert the fraction $\frac{5}{8}$ to a decimal.

Q22 Convert the fraction $\frac{7}{80}$ to a decimal.

Q23 Express 0.82 as a percentage.

Q24 Express 0.345 as a percentage.

Q25 Express 30% as a fraction in its lowest terms.

Q26 Express 0.3% as a fraction in its lowest terms.

Q27 Express $\frac{7}{8}$ as a percentage.

Q28 Express $\frac{6}{25}$ as a percentage.

Questions 29 to 33 can be worked out using the 'spotting' methods.

Q29 Find the missing value x from the pair of proportional sets:

8   x 20
2   4   5

Q30 Find the missing number y from the pair of proportional sets:

25   30
y 6

Q31 Find the missing number z from the pair of proportional sets:

21   z
7   30

Q32 Find the missing number *x* from the pair of proportional sets:

81   18

x   2

Q33 Find the missing number *y* from the pair of proportional sets:

y   21

8   24

Q34 Find the missing number *z* from the pair of proportional sets:

4   10

10   *z*

Q35 Find the missing number *x* from the pair of proportional sets:

x   10

7   35

Q36 Find the missing number *y* from the pair of proportional sets:

32   *y*

19   41

Give your answer correct to two significant figures (see Chapter 12).

Q37 Find the missing number *z* from the pair of proportional sets:

225   420

192   *z*

Give your answer correct to three significant figures (see Chapter 12).

Q38 Find the missing number *x* from the pair of proportional sets:

x   11.3

22.5   15.7

Give your answer correct to three significant figures (see Chapter 12).

A1 Not proportional.

A2 Proportional. Each value of the lower set is four times the corresponding value of the upper set.

A3 Not proportional.

A4 Proportional. Each number of the lower set is 2.5 times the corresponding value of the upper set.

A5 Proportional. Each value of the upper set is 5 times the corresponding value of the lower set.

A6 Proportional. Each value of the lower set is 1.5 times the corresponding value of the upper set.

A7 $\dfrac{63}{72}$

A8 $\dfrac{28}{49}$

A9 $\dfrac{26}{117}$

A10 $\dfrac{3}{5}$

A11 $\dfrac{1}{5}$

A12 $\dfrac{7}{9}$

A13 $\dfrac{3}{5}$

A14 $\dfrac{20}{7} = 2\dfrac{6}{7}$

A15 $\dfrac{15}{13}$

A16 $\dfrac{12}{17}$

A17 $\dfrac{35}{9} = 3\dfrac{8}{9}$

A18 $\dfrac{4}{5}$

A19 $\dfrac{87}{100}$

A20 $\dfrac{7}{8}$

A21 0.625

A22 0.0875

A23 82%

A24 34.5%

A25 $\dfrac{3}{10}$

A26 $\dfrac{3}{1000}$

A27 87.5%

A28 24%

A29 16

A30 5

A31 90

A32 9

A33 7

A34 25

A35 2

A36 69

A37 358

A38 16.2

3

Systems of units

Learning objectives

By the end of this chapter you will be able to:

- express a mass, volume or length in different metric units
- convert a mass, length or volume from the imperial measure to the SI equivalent
- find the temperature in Celsius of a temperature expressed as Fahrenheit

Mass and weight

Mass is the measure of quantity of matter. The Système International (SI) unit of mass is the kilogram (kg).

Weight is a force. The SI unit of force is the newton (N). A particle of mass 1 kg is attracted towards the centre of the earth by a force of g newtons, where g is the acceleration due to gravity and has a value that varies slightly at different points on the earth's surface. The value of g is about $9.8 \, \text{m/s}^2$, so a mass of 1 kg has a weight of about 9.8 newtons.

In everyday life the word 'weight' is often used instead of the word 'mass'. A person's weight is stated as being, say, 160 kg and the units indicate that mass rather than force is implied. In pharmacy, 'weight' is traditionally used in cases where 'mass' would be more appropriate and where it is obvious from the context and perhaps from the units, that a force is not intended. For example, tables of body weights are used and in the *British Pharmacopoeia* concentration ratios are stated as being w/v or w/w, i.e. weight in volume and weight in weight. In each case it is mass rather than weight that is being considered.

Rather than always using the correct term 'mass' in this book, 'weight' is used to conform with current pharmacy texts. No forces are used, so whenever 'weight' occurs, 'mass' is implied.

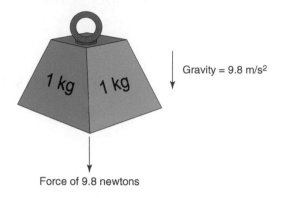

Force of 9.8 newtons

Metric units

The units most commonly used in pharmacy are those of volume and mass. The basic metric unit of volume is the litre (L or l) and the basic metric unit of mass is the gram (g). (The litre is also the SI unit of volume, but the SI unit of mass is the kilogram (kg).)

Prefixes are used to indicate multiples and submultiples of units. Those in general use are shown in Table 3.1 (see also Appendix 1). Thus, for the basic unit of the litre, one thousand litres are equal to 1 kL and one-thousandth of a litre is 1 mL. For the basic unit of the gram, one thousand grams are equal to 1 kg and one-thousandth of a gram is 1 mg.

In this book the only units we use with prefixes are kg, mg, kL and mL. For other multiples or submultiples we write the word in full (e.g. microlitre, microgram, megagram).

The metric system is based on the decimal system (see p. 11) so, as with decimals, we have a system of 'place values'. Instead of column headings of units, hundreds, thousands, etc. we have the following.

Table 3.1 Common prefixes

Prefix	mega	kilo	milli	micro
Factor	10^6	10^3	10^{-3}	10^{-6}
Symbol	M	k	m	μ

Mass

megagrams –   – kg –   – g –   –   mg –   –   micrograms
Factors 10^6 10^5 10^4 10^3 10^2 10^1 1 10^{-1} 10^{-2} 10^{-3} 10^{-4} 10^{-5} 10^{-6}

Volume

megalitres –   – kL –   – L –   –   mL –   –   microlitres

There are other metric prefixes for some of the headings that we have denoted by dashes, such as decigram and centigram, but we will not make use of them here (see Appendix 1).

Changing metric units

We can make use of 'place values' in changing metric units. Tackling the task in this way should avoid mistakes such as multiplying by a power of ten when division should have been carried out, or vice versa.

Example 3.1

Change 200 mg to grams.

First write down column headings involving the relevant units and underneath enter the 200 with the unit digit (the last zero) in the mg column. Fill the empty columns with zeroes. The value in grams is read off by placing a decimal point after the digit in the grams column, i.e.

	g	–	–	mg	
200 mg =	0	2	0	0	= 0.2 g

Example 3.2

Convert 5473 mL to litres.

	L	–	–	mL	
5473 mL =	5	4	7	3	= 5.473 L

Example 3.3

Convert *1.26 mg to micrograms.*

	mg	–	–	micrograms	
1.26 mg =	1	2	6	0	= 1260 micrograms

Example 3.4

Convert *135 465 micrograms to grams.*

	g	–	–	mg	–	–	micrograms	
135 465 micrograms =	0	1	3	5	4	6	5	= 0.135 465 g

Example 3.5

Convert *0.003 745 kL to mL.*

	kL	–	–	L	–	–	mL	
0.003 745 kL =	0	0	0	3	7	4	5	= 3745 mL

Table 3.2 may be useful to convert numbers, as above.

Changing units between different systems of measurement

Units of measurement such as feet and inches, gallons and pints and stones and pounds are still in everyday use. It may therefore be necessary to convert measurements between these systems and the metric system.

Table 3.2 Place values

Prefix	mega			kilo	hector				deci	centi	milli			micro
Length				kilometre (km)			metre (m)			centimetre (cm)	millimetre (mm)			micrometre (μm)
Weight				kilogram (kg)			gram (g)				milligram (mg)			microgram (μg)
Volume							litre (L)				millilitre (mL)			
Moles							mole (mol)				millimole (mmol)			micromole (μmol)
Factor	10^6	10^5	10^4	10^3	10^2	10^1	1	10^{-1}	10^{-2}	10^{-3}		10^{-4}	10^{-5}	10^{-6}
Convert 56 kg to grams			5	6	0	0	0				Answer: 56 000 g			

Proportional sets can be used to aid the conversion. The relevant conversion factor must be found (see Appendix 2 for a list of common conversion factors) and used in the proportional sets, as in Example 3.6.

Example 3.6

Convert 3.4 pints to litres.

The conversion factor between the two sets of measurements is $1 L = 1.76$ pints. Let the required number of litres be x. Setting up proportional sets:

litres	x	1
pints	3.4	1.76

Corresponding pairs are in the same ratio:

$$\frac{x}{3.4} = \frac{1}{1.76}$$

$$x = \frac{3.4}{1.76} = 1.93$$

$$3.4 \text{ pints} = 1.93 \text{ L}$$

Note: replacing the value for x in the proportional set allows us to check relative values and so avoid errors.

Body-weight tables sometimes use weight in kilograms. In fact, to calculate a person's BMI (Body Mass Index) you need to know their height in metres and their weight in kilograms as the equation for this calculation is:

$$\text{BMI} = \frac{\text{weight (kg)}}{\text{height}^2 \text{(m)}} \quad \text{or} \quad \frac{\text{weight (kg)}}{\text{height} \times \text{height(m)}}$$

Most people know their weight only in stones and pounds and their height in feet and inches. It is therefore necessary to be able to convert values from one set of units to the other.

Example 3.7

Convert 106.4 kg to stones and pounds.

Conversion factor: 1 pound = 0.4536 kg.

Let the required number of pounds be *y*. Setting up proportional sets:

pounds	*y*	1
kilograms	106.4	4536

$$\frac{y}{106.4} = \frac{1}{0.4536}$$
$$y = \frac{106.4}{0.4536} = 234.56$$

106.4 kg is equal to 235 pounds (to the nearest pound). There are 14 pounds in 1 stone, so 235 pounds = 16 stone 11 pounds.

Example 3.8

Convert 10 stone 4 pounds to kilograms.

Conversion factor: 1 pound = 0.4536 kg.

14 pounds = 1 stone, so 10 stone 4 pounds = 144 pounds.

Let the required number of kilograms be *x*. Setting up proportional sets:

pounds	1	144
kilograms	0.4536	*x*

Corresponding pairs are in the same ratio:

$$\frac{x}{144} = \frac{0.4536}{1}$$
$$x = 144 \times 0.4536 = 65.3$$

10 stone 4 pounds = 65.3 kg.

Example 3.9

Convert 5 feet 10 inches into metres.

Conversion factor: 1 inch = 25.4 mm = 0.0254 m

12 inches = 1 foot, so 5 feet 10 inches = 70 inches.

Let the required number of metres be x. Setting up proportional sets:

inches   1   70

metres   0.0254 x

Corresponding pairs are in the same ratio:

$$\frac{x}{70} = \frac{0.254}{1}$$
$$x = 70 \times 0.0254 = 1.778$$

5 feet 10 inches = 1.778 m.

Using these conversions the BMI can be calculated by fitting the numbers into the equation.

Example 3.10

What would be the BMI for a patient who weighs 10 stone and 4 pounds and is 5 feet 10 inches tall?

From Example 3.8: 10 stone 4 pounds = 65.3 kg.

From Example 3.9: 5 feet 10 inches = 1.778 m.

$$BMI = \frac{weight\ (kg)}{height^2(m)} = \frac{65.3}{(1.778)^2} = \frac{65.3}{1.778 \times 1.778}$$

Therefore, the BMI = 20.7.

Conversions of temperature between degrees Fahrenheit and degrees Celsius

If we are given the information that 50 degrees Celsius = 122 degrees Fahrenheit, then to find the number of degrees Celsius (y) corresponding to 95 degrees Fahrenheit we may be tempted to set up sets of corresponding values:

degrees Celsius	50	y
degrees Fahrenheit	122	95

but beware: 75 degrees Celsius = 167 degrees Fahrenheit, so if we write sets of the two known corresponding pairs:

degrees Celsius	50	75
degrees Fahrenheit	122	167

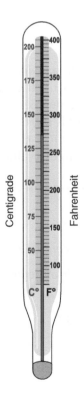

we can see that the two sets are not proportional and therefore, we cannot equate ratios of corresponding pairs.

The freezing point of water is 0 degrees Celsius and 32 degrees Fahrenheit, so if we subtract 32 from Fahrenheit values we should then get a pair of proportional sets:

| degrees Celsius | 50 | 75 |
| degrees Fahrenheit minus 32 | 90 | 135 |

$90 = 50$ times 1.8 and $135 = 75$ times 1.8. The sets are proportional.

Returning to the task of finding the number of degrees Celsius (y) corresponding to 95 degrees Fahrenheit:

| degrees Celsius | 50 | y |
| degrees Fahrenheit minus 32 | 122-32 | 95-32 |

$$\frac{y}{63} = \frac{50}{90}$$
$$y = \frac{63 \times 50}{90} = 35$$

95 degrees Fahrenheit = 35 degrees Celsius.

Do not assume that all sets of corresponding values are proportional.

The boiling point of water on the Celsius scale is 100 degrees and on the Fahrenheit scale is 212 degrees, so the range of values between freezing point and boiling point is 100 degrees on the Celsius scale and 180 degrees on the Fahrenheit scale. It is therefore useful to use these ranges as corresponding values in changing values from one scale to the other.

Example 3.11

Change 25 degrees Celsius to degrees Fahrenheit.

Let the corresponding number of degrees Fahrenheit be x. Setting up proportional sets:

| degrees Fahrenheit minus 32 | 180 | x – 32 |
| degrees Celsius | 100 | 25 |

$\rightarrow$

Corresponding pairs are in the same ratio.

We can spot that 100 divided by 4 is 25, so 180 divided by 4 will be $x - 32$, therefore:

$$x - 32 = 45$$

$$x = 45 + 32 = 77$$

25 degrees Celsius = 77 degrees Fahrenheit.

Example 3.12

Change 68 degrees Fahrenheit to degrees Celsius.

Let the required number of degrees Celsius be y. Setting up proportional sets:

degrees Fahrenheit minus 32	180	68 – 32
degrees Celsius	100	y

Corresponding pairs are in the same ratio:

$$\frac{y}{36} = \frac{100}{180}$$

$$y = \frac{100 \times 36}{180} = 20$$

68 degrees Fahrenheit = 20 degrees Celsius.

Conversion of units

Practice calculations

Answers are given at the end of the chapter.

Q1   Change 0.035 g to milligrams.

Q2   Change 1384 mg to grams.

Q3   Change 437 mL to litres.

Q4 Change 12.47 L to millilitres.

Q5 Change 0.87 mL to microlitres.

Q6 Change 15 750 microlitres to millilitres.

Q7 Change 0.0025 kg to grams.

Q8 Change 12 g to kilograms.

Q9 Change 0.72 megalitres to kilolitres.

Q10 Change 145 kg to megagrams.

Q11 Use the conversion factor 1 L = 1.76 pints to express:
(a) 6.43 pints in litres
(b) 2.42 L in pints.

Q12 Use the conversion factor 1 pound = 0.4536 kg to express:
(a) 9 stones 4 pounds in kilograms (1 stone = 14 pounds)
(b) 49 kg in stones and pounds.

Q13 the boiling point of water is 100 degrees Celsius or 212 degrees Fahrenheit. The freezing point of water is 0 degrees Celsius or 32 degrees Fahrenheit. Express:
(a) 15 degrees Celsius in degrees Fahrenheit (to the nearest degree)
(b) 88 degrees Fahrenheit in degrees Celsius (to the nearest degree).

Answers

A1	35 mg	**A5**	870 microlitres
A2	1.384 g	**A6**	15.75 mL
A3	0.437 L	**A7**	2.5 g
A4	12 470 mL	**A8**	0.012 kg

A9   720 kL

A10   0.145 megagrams

A11   (a) 3.65 L
           (b) 4.26 pints

A12   (a) 59 kg
           (b) 7 stone 10 pounds

A13   (a) 59 degrees Fahrenheit
           (b) 31 degrees Celsius

4

Concentrations

Learning objectives

By the end of this chapter you will be able to:

- state the relationship between the different methods of expressing the concentration of a pharmaceutical preparation
- convert one expression of concentration to another
- calculate the amount of ingredient required to make a product of a stated strength

Introduction

Pharmaceutical preparations consist of a number of different ingredients in a vehicle to produce a product. The ingredients and vehicles used in a product can be solid, liquid or gas.

Concentration is an expression of the ratio of the amount of an ingredient to the amount of product. It can be expressed in several ways:

- In the case of a solid ingredient in a liquid vehicle the ratio is expressed as a weight in volume, denoted by w/v (for example sugar granules dissolved in a cup of coffee)
- For a liquid ingredient in a solid vehicle the ratio is expressed as a volume in weight, denoted by v/w (for example lemon juice drizzled on the top of a cake)
- If both ingredient and vehicle are liquids the ratio is expressed as a volume in volume, denoted by v/v (for example milk added to a cup of coffee)
- When the ingredient and vehicle are both solid the ratio is expressed as a weight in weight, denoted by w/w (for example the blueberries as a proportion of the whole blueberry muffin)

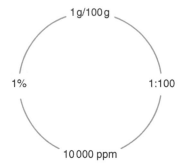

- The concentration of pharmaceutical preparations usually describes the strength of the drug in the preparations. In practice it is important that the patient receives the correct amount of the drug
- If a patient receives too much of the drug they are likely to experience side-effects; side-effects are often dose-related, so the higher the amount of the drug the stronger the side-effect
- If a patient receives too little of the drug, then their treatment is likely to be less effective than the prescriber intended. This can lead to a deterioration in the health of the patient.

We know that rational numbers can be expressed as ratios, fractions, decimals or percentages. As concentrations are expressions of ratios, they can also be expressed in different forms. The forms traditionally used are those of amount strengths, ratio strengths, parts per million and percentage strength.

Each of these four forms can be expressions of w/w, v/v, w/v or v/w, depending on whether solids or liquids are involved.

For ratio strengths, parts per million and percentage strengths in w/w or v/v the amounts of ingredients and product must be expressed in the same units:

- a ratio of 7 mL to 12 mL is the ratio 7 : 12 v/v
- a ratio of 3 mg to 5 mg is the ratio 3 : 5 w/w.

As long as the units used are the same, they lead to the same ratio.

For a concentration of 3 mg to 5 g, we need to change to the same units before we can express the w/w ratio.

Converting 5 g to milligrams:

$$
\begin{array}{ccccc}
\text{g} & - & - & \text{mg} & \\
5\,\text{g} = \quad 5 & 0 & 0 & 0 & = 5000\,\text{mg}
\end{array}
$$

The ratio becomes 3 mg to 5000 mg, which is the ratio 3 : 5000 w/w.

In the case of w/v and v/w there is an agreed convention that states that weight is expressed in grams and volume is expressed in millilitres.

Let us now examine each of the traditional ways of expressing concentrations in more detail.

Amount strengths

Amount strengths can appear in any of the four forms, w/w, v/v, w/v or v/w. The amount strength is a ratio of the quantities and any units can be used, i.e. g/mL, mg/mL, mg/g, mL/mL, g/g, g/mL, etc. The units are stated in all cases.

Keep out of the reach and sight of children		
100 g Menthol 1% w/w in aqueous cream		
Apply as directed		
For external use only		
Mrs A Patient		08.01.15
The Pharmacy 2 The Road, The Town 0123 45678	Disp	Chkd

Let us first consider a solid dissolved in a liquid to produce a solution.

Example 4.1

A preparation contains 900 mg of sodium chloride dissolved in water to produce 100 mL of solution. Express the concentration of the solution as an amount strength.

The concentration of this solution can be expressed as an amount strength in units of mg/100 mL, mg/mL, g/100 mL, g/L and so on.

To convert the above concentration of sodium chloride solution into these different representations we use proportional sets. The solution contains the same concentration of sodium chloride irrespective of whether we have 100 mL, 50 mL or 1 mL. The ratio of sodium chloride to product is constant.

Let us consider how the concentration could be expressed as the ratio mg/mL and as the ratio g/mL.

(continued)

Let the number of milligrams of sodium chloride in 1 mL of water be z. Setting up proportional sets:

sodium chloride (mg)	900	z
water (mL) to	100	1

The reason that we write *to* 100 mL rather than *in* 100 mL is that the sodium chloride is dissolved in water and made up to 100 mL with water; 900 mg of sodium chloride and 100 mL of water will produce more than 100 mL of solution, so the amount of water required to make 100 mL of solution will be less than 100 mL because of the displacement caused by the sodium chloride. We consider the concept of displacement and displacement values later. In addition, some drugs, such as strong concentrations of alcohol, may cause a contraction in volume when dissolved in water. For this reason, in pharmacy we always make up *to* volume.

From the proportional sets, it can be spotted that $z=9$, so the concentration of sodium chloride in this solution can be represented by an amount strength of 9 mg/mL.

Sodium chloride in water is a solid in a liquid and is therefore expressed as milligrams (a weight) in millilitres (a volume). This is a w/v ratio. We can also convert 9 mg to grams:

g	–	–	mg	
9 mg =	0 0 0		9	= 0.009 g

The concentration of sodium chloride, which was earlier expressed as 9 mg/mL, can therefore also be represented by an amount strength of 0.009 g/mL.

Ratio strengths

Ratio strength is expressed as a ratio in the form 1 in r. The corresponding fraction would have a numerator of 1.

The agreed convention states that, when ratio strength represents a solid in a liquid involving units of weight and volume, the weight is expressed in grams and the volume in millilitres.

1 in 500 potassium permanganate in water is a solid in a liquid and is therefore a weight in volume (w/v) ratio strength. This means that the solution contains 1 g of potassium permanganate made up to 500 mL with water.

Example 4.2

---

2 L of an aqueous solution contains 50 mL of ethanol. Express this as a ratio strength.

As this solution is a volume in volume we need to convert to the same units before we can express this as a ratio.
Converting 2 L into millilitres:

$$L \quad - \quad - \quad mL$$
$$2 L = \quad 2 \quad 0 \quad 0 \quad 0 \quad = 2000 \, mL$$

Let the volume of product in millilitres containing 1 mL of ethanol be r.
Setting up proportional sets:

ethanol (mL)   50   1

product (mL)   2000 r

By 'spotting', $r = 40$, so the ratio strength is 1 in 40 v/v.

Example 4.3 illustrates the calculation of a ratio strength for a solid in a solid.

Example 4.3

---

5 g of product contains 250 mg of sulfur in yellow soft paraffin. Express this as a ratio strength.

This is a weight in weight product because both the sulfur and the yellow soft paraffin are solid. The weights must be converted to the same units before the concentration can be stated as a ratio strength.
Converting 250 mg to grams:

$$g \quad - \quad - \quad mg$$
$$250 \, mg = \quad 0 \quad 2 \quad 5 \quad 0 \quad = 0.25 \, g$$

(continued)

Let the weight in grams of product containing 1 g of sulfur be r. Setting up proportional sets:

sulfur (g)   0.25   1

product (g)   5 r

Corresponding pairs are in the same ratio, therefore:

$$\frac{5}{0.25} = \frac{r}{1}$$

Solving for the unknown:

$$r = \frac{5}{0.25}$$

$$r = 20$$

The ratio strength is 1 in 20 w/w.

Parts per million

Parts per million (ppm) is used to denote concentrations in cases when the ratio of ingredient to product is very small. It is equivalent to a ratio in the form of p in 1000 000 or a fraction in which the denominator is 1000 000.

By the agreed convention, 1 ppm weight in volume is 1 g in 1000 000 mL; 1 ppm weight in weight is 1 mg per 1000 000 mg or 1 g per 1000 000 g. In volume in volume it is 1 mL in 1000 000 mL or 1 L in 1000 000 L.

Example 4.4

Fluoride in a water supply is expressed as parts per million w/v. Fluoride supplements should not be taken if the amount of fluoride in the water supply exceeds 0.7 parts per million w/v according to the British National Formulary (BNF). *Express this ratio in mg/L.*

By convention, 0.7 ppm can be represented as 0.7 g in 1000 000 mL.

$\rightarrow$

Converting 0.7 g to milligrams:

g   –   –   mg

0.7 g =   0   7   0   0   = 700 mg

Converting 1 000 000 mL into litres:

L   –   –   mL

1 000 000 mL =   1   0   0   0   0   0   0   = 1000 L

0.7 ppm w/v = 700 mg per 1000 L = 0.7 mg/L.
Therefore, it can be seen that part per million is the same as mg/L. These representations of the concentrations of fluoride appear to be used interchangeably in documentation. In the BNF fluoride levels are expressed as ppm and micrograms/L.

Example 4.5

If the concentration of fluoride is 0.25 ppm w/v, how many litres would contain 1 mg of fluoride?

0.25 ppm w/v means 0.25 g per 1 000 000 mL.
Converting 0.25 g to milligrams:

g   –   –   mg

0.25 g =   0   2   5   0   = 250 mg

Let the amount of product in millilitres containing 1 mg of fluoride be y. Setting up proportional sets:

fluoride (mg)   250   1

product (mL)   1 000 000 y

Corresponding pairs of values are in the same ratio so:

$$\frac{1000\ 000}{250} = \frac{y}{1}$$

(continued)

Solving for the unknown in the proportional sets:

$$y = \frac{1000\ 000}{250}$$

$$y = 4000$$

Hence 4000 mL contains 1 mg of fluoride.
Converting 4000 mL to litres:

	L	–	–	mL	
4000 mL =	4	0	0	0	= 4 L

4 L therefore contains 1 mg of fluoride.

Percentage concentration

In terms of parts, a percentage is the amount of ingredient in 100 parts of the product. In the w/v and v/w cases, using the convention, the units are grams per 100 mL and millilitres per 100 g.

Example 4.6

A cream contains 12 g of drug X made up to 100 g with cream base. What is the percentage concentration?

From the information above the percentage concentration is the units in grams in 100 g.

As the amount in grams is 12 g in 100 g, it is 12% w/w.

Example 4.7

Express 1 in 500 w/v solution of potassium permanganate as a percentage.

Let the number of grams of potassium permanganate in 100 mL of product be x. Setting up proportional sets:

$\rightarrow$

potassium permanganate (g)   1 x

product (mL)   500   100

We can spot that we divide 500 by 5 to get 100, so we divide 1 by 5 to get $\frac{1}{5}$ and therefore $x = 0.2$ and the percentage of potassium permanganate is 0.2% w/v.

Example 4.8

Express 900 mg of sodium chloride made up to 100 mL with water as a percentage.

To express the value as a percentage, we need to convert the number of milligrams in 100 mL to grams in 100 mL:

	g	–	–	mg	
900 mg =	0	9	0	0	= 0.9 g

There is 0.9 g of sodium chloride in 100 mL of solution. The percentage is 0.9% w/v.

Example 4.9

A morphine sulfate injection contains 10 mg/mL. What is the percentage concentration?

To express the value as a percentage, we need to convert the number of milligrams in 1 mL to grams in 100 mL:

	g	–	–	mg	
10 mg =	0	0	1	0	= 0.01 g

There is 0.01 g of morphine sulfate in 1 mL of solution.

Which means that there is $0.01 \times 100\,g = 1\,g$ in 100 mL.

The percentage is 1% w/v.

Converting expressions of concentration from one form to another

Let us consider a general case. Let the amount of the ingredient be *a* and the amount of product be *b*. Let *p* be the amount in 100 parts (the percentage concentration), 1 in *r* be the ratio strength and *m* be the number of parts per million.

We can set up the following proportional sets:

	amount	percentage	ratio strength	ppm
ingredient	*a*	*p*	1	*m*
product	*b*	100	*r*	1 000 000

This table shows the relationship between the different expressions of concentration. By using the proportional sets of the known expression of concentration and the required expression of concentration, it is possible to convert from one expression to another.

Example 4.10

A solution contains 20 mL of ethanol in 500 mL of product. Express the concentration as a ratio strength and as a percentage strength.

Let *p* be the percentage strength and let the ratio strength be 1 in *r*. Setting up proportional sets as above:

	volume	ratio	percentage
ethanol (mL)	20	1	*p*
product (mL)	500	*r*	100

Corresponding pairs of values are in the same ratio so:

$$\frac{500}{20} = \frac{r}{1}$$

Solving for the unknown in the proportional sets:

$$r = \frac{500}{20}$$

$$r = 25$$

→

By 'spotting' we can see that $p = \frac{20}{5} = 4$, so the mixture can be expressed as the ratio strength 1 in 25 v/v or as the percentage strength 4% v/v.

Example 4.11

A solid ingredient mixed with a solid vehicle has a ratio strength of 1 in 40. Find the percentage strength and the amount strength expressed as grams per gram.

Let p represent the percentage strength and let a grams be the weight of ingredient in 1 g of product. Setting up proportional sets:

	ratio strength	percentage	amount strength (g/g)
ingredient (g)	1	p	a
product (g)	40	100	1

Corresponding pairs of values are in the same ratio so:

$$\frac{1}{40} = \frac{p}{100}$$

Solving for the unknown in the proportional sets:

$$p = \frac{100}{40}$$

$$p = 2.5$$

Corresponding pairs of values are in the same ratio so:

$$\frac{1}{40} = \frac{a}{1}$$

Solving for the unknown in the proportional sets:

$$a = 0.025$$

The concentration of the mixture can be expressed as either 2.5% w/w or 0.025 g/g.

Example 4.12

A solution contains a solid dissolved in a liquid. The ratio strength is 1 in 2000 w/v. What are the percentage strength and the amount concentration expressed as mg/mL?

By convention, a ratio strength 1: 2000 w/v means 1 g in 2000 mL and the percentage strength is the number of grams of ingredient in 100 mL of product.

Let the percentage strength be *p* and the amount of solid in grams in 1 mL of product be *a*. Setting up proportional sets:

	ratio	percentage	amount strength (g/mL)
solid (g)	1	p	a
product (mL)	2000	100	1

Corresponding pairs of values are in the same ratio so:

$$\frac{1}{2000} = \frac{p}{100}$$

Solving for the unknown in the proportional sets:

$$p = \frac{100}{2000}$$
$$p = 0.05$$

Corresponding pairs of values are in the same ratio so:

$$\frac{1}{2000} = \frac{a}{1}$$

Solving for the unknown in the proportional sets:

$$a = \frac{1}{2000}$$
$$a = 0.0005\,g$$

$\rightarrow$

Converting 0.0005 g to milligrams:

$$
\begin{array}{cccccc}
g & - & - & & mg & \\
0.0005\,g = & 0 \quad 0 & 0 \quad 0 & 5 & = 0.5\,mg
\end{array}
$$

The concentration of 1 in 2000 w/v can be expressed as 0.05% w/v or 0.5 mg/mL.

Example 4.13

A liquid ingredient mixed with another liquid vehicle has a concentration of 5% v/v. Find the ratio strength and the amount strength expressed as mL/mL.

5% v/v can be expressed as 5 mL of ingredient in 100 mL of product.
    Let the ratio strength be 1 in r and the amount of ingredient in millilitres in 1 mL of product be a. Setting up proportional sets:

	percentage	ratio	amount strength (mL/mL)
ingredient (mL)	5	1	a
product (mL)	100	r	1

By 'spotting' we can see that:

$$r = \frac{100}{5} = 20$$

$$a = \frac{5}{100} = 0.05$$

The ratio is 1 in 20 v/v and the amount strength in mL/mL is 0.05 mL/mL.

Example 4.14

5 g of solid ingredient is added to 45 g of a base. Find the percentage strength, the ratio strength and the amount strength expressed as g/g.
                                                                    (continued)

Remember that for weight in weight and volume in volume the product is equal to the sum of the vehicle and the ingredient, in this case $5 + 45 = 50\,g$.

Let p be the percentage strength, 1 in r be the ratio strength and a grams be the amount in 1 g of product. Setting up proportional sets:

	amount	percentage	ratio	amount strength (g/g)
ingredient (g)	5	p	1	a
product (g)	50	100	r	1

By 'spotting' we can see that:

$$p = \left(\frac{5}{50} \times 100 \right) = 10$$

$$r = \left(\frac{50}{5} \times 1 \right) = 10$$

$$a = \left(\frac{5}{50} \times 1 \right) = 0.1$$

The concentration can therefore be expressed as 10% w/w or 1 in 10 w/w or 0.1 g/g.

Calculating the amount of ingredient required to make up a percentage solution

In the same way as converting from one expression of concentration to another, it is also possible to use the proportional sets to calculate the amount of ingredient required to produce a known amount of a known percentage product.

This can be achieved by using the following proportional sets:

	amount	percentage
ingredient	a	p
product	b	100

Values p and b will be known and, therefore, a can be calculated.

Example 4.15

How many milligrams of aluminium acetate are required to prepare 500 mL of a 0.03% w/v solution?

Aluminium acetate is a solid and is expressed as a weight, in this case milligrams. The vehicle is a liquid and is expressed in millilitres. By convention 0.03% w/v means 0.03 g in 100 mL so each 100 mL contains 0.03 g of aluminium acetate.

Converting 0.03 g to milligrams:

$$g \quad - \quad - \quad mg$$

$$0.03\,g = \quad 0 \quad 0 \quad 3 \quad 0 \quad = 30\,mg$$

Let x be the number of milligrams of aluminium acetate in 500 mL. Setting up proportional sets:

aluminium acetate (mg)	x	30
product (mL)	500	100

By 'spotting' it can be seen that:

$$x = 30 \times 5 = 150$$

150 mg of aluminium acetate is required to produce 500 mL of a 0.03% w/v solution.

Calculating the amount of ingredient required to prepare a ratio strength solution

When the final concentration of the product is expressed as a ratio strength, the following proportional sets can be used to calculate the amount of ingredient to produce a known amount of product.

	amount	ratio
ingredient	a	1
product	b	r

In this situation, r and b will be known and a will be calculated.

Example 4.16

What is the amount of potassium permanganate in 300 mL of a 1 in 25 solution and what is the percentage strength of the solution?

By convention, a ratio strength of 1 in 25 means 1 g in 25 mL.

Let a be the number of grams of potassium permanganate in 300 mL and p be the percentage strength. Setting up proportional sets:

	ratio	amount in 300 mL	percentage
potassium permanganate (g)	1	a	p
product (mL)	25	300	100

Corresponding pairs are in the same ratio:

$$\frac{a}{300} = \frac{1}{25}$$

Solving for the unknown:

$$a = \frac{1 \times 300}{25} = 12$$

Amount of potassium permanganate $= 12$ g.

By 'spotting' we can see that:

$$p = 4$$

The solution therefore contains 4 g potassium permanganate in 100 mL $= 4\%$ w/v.

There are 12 g of potassium permanganate in 300 mL of solution and the percentage strength is 4% w/v.

Representation of concentrations

Answers are given at the end of the chapter.

Q1   Convert the following ratio strengths into percentage strengths:

   (a)   1 in 25

   (b)   1 in 20

(c)   1 in 50

(d)   1 in 800

(e)   1 in 500

(f)   1 in 2000

(g)   1 in 300

Q2   What is the concentration of the solutions, expressed as percentage strength and ratio strength, when the following amounts of drug Z are dissolved in enough water to produce 125 mL of solution?

(a)   25 g

(b)   50 g

(c)   60 g

(d)   5 g

(e)   7 g

Q3   If the following amounts of drug are made up to 5 g with lactose what is the percentage concentration of the resulting mix?

(a)   100 mg

(b)   150 mg

(c)   200 mg

(d)   300 mg

(e)   500 mg

Q4   How many milligrams of y are needed to make 200 mL of a 1 in 500 solution?

Q5   How many millilitres of y are needed to produce 400 mL of a 1 in 200 solution?

Q6   How many milligrams of y are needed to produce 25 g of a 1 in 5 ointment?

Q7   How many grams of y are there in 250 mL of a 1 in 80 solution?

Q8   Potassium permanganate   0.1 g

Purified water to   100 mL

How many millilitres of a 2.5% potassium permanganate solution could be used in place of the 0.1 g in the above formula?

Q9   How many milligrams of x are needed to make 5 mL of an 8% solution?

Q10   How many millilitres of x are needed to make 600 mL of a 3% solution?

Q11   How many milligrams of x are needed to make 200 mL of a 3.4% solution?

Q12   How many milligrams of x are there in 100 mL of a 0.01% solution?

Q13   How much calamine is required to produce 250 g of a 3% ointment?

Q14   What volume of 17% w/v solution contains 1.5 g of ingredient?

Q15   What volume of 20% w/v solution contains 5 g of ingredient?

Q16   What volume of 15% w/v solution contains 7 g of ingredient?

Q17   What volume of 34% w/v solution contains 150 g of ingredient?

Answers

A1 (a) 4%
    (b) 5%
    (c) 2%
    (d) 0.125%
    (e) 0.2%
    (f) 0.05%
    (g) 0.33%

A2 (a) 20%, 1 in 5
    (b) 40%, 1 in 2.5
    (c) 48%, 1 in 2.1
    (d) 4%, 1 in 25
    (e) 5.6%, 1 in 17.9

A3 (a) 2%
    (b) 3%
    (c) 4%
    (d) 6%
    (e) 10%

A4   400 mg

A5   2 mL

A6   5000 mg

A7   3.1 g

A8 4 mL

A9 400 mg

A10 18 mL

A11 6800 mg

A12 10 mg

A13 7.5 g

A14 8.8 mL

A15 25 mL

A16 46.7 mL

A17 441.2 mL

5

Dilutions

Learning objectives

By the end of this chapter you will be able to:

- calculate the final strength of a diluted product
- calculate the amount of ingredient in a product which is then diluted to a stated strength
- calculate the volume of concentrated waters (e.g. chloroform water) required to make different volumes of single- and double-strength concentrations
- understand and calculate triturations of solids and liquids
- calculate the ratios in which two products must be mixed to produce a given concentration

Simple dilutions

When a product is diluted there is a change in the amount of product, although at the same time the amount of ingredient in the product remains the same.

In practice, a pharmaceutical product may be supplied in a concentrated form. This has many advantages as the product may be more stable in the concentrated form, it takes up less space in the pharmacy and, most importantly, the pharmacist can then dilute the preparation to produce several different final strengths of product. However, failure by the pharmacist to correctly calculate the dilution will result in the patient receiving too much or too little of the active ingredient.

If a solution containing 5 g of an ingredient in 200 mL of product is diluted to 400 mL with vehicle, the final product becomes 400 mL containing 5 g of ingredient. The volume of product has changed (it has doubled) and the amount of ingredient is still 5 g.

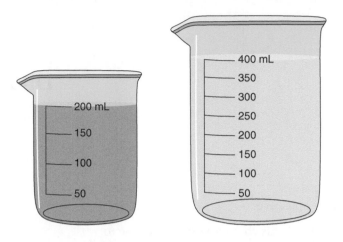

The amount strength has therefore changed from 5 g/200 mL to 5 g/400 mL.

Example 5.1

A product consists of a solid ingredient in a solid vehicle; 2 g of the solid ingredient is contained in 500 g of product. A further 250 g of vehicle is added to the product. Find the concentration of the diluted mixture as a percentage strength, a ratio strength and an amount strength in mg/g.

The amount of the ingredient will remain the same, i.e. 2 g. The total amount of product will change to 750 g:

	amount	percentage	ratio	amount strength (g/g)
ingredient (g)	2	p	1	a
product (g)	750	100	r	1

By setting up proportional sets and solving equations, or by 'spotting', we get:

$p = 0.27$

$r = 375$

$a = 0.0027$

→

Converting 0.0027 g to milligrams:

$$\begin{array}{ccccccc} g & - & - & & mg & & \\ 0.0027\,g = & 0 & 0 & 0 & 2 & 7 & = 2.7\,mg \end{array}$$

The diluted product has a percentage strength of 0.27% w/w, a ratio strength of 1 in 375 w/w and an amount strength of 2.7 mg/g.

Example 5.2 shows the method of calculating the final concentration of the diluted product starting with a ratio strength.

Example 5.2

100 mL of a 1 in 50 w/v solution is diluted to 1000 mL. Find the concentration of the diluted product as a percentage strength, a ratio strength and an amount strength expressed as mg/mL.

By convention, 1 in 50 means 1 g in 50 mL.
 Let the number of grams of ingredient in 100 mL of product be g. Setting up proportional sets:

ingredient (g)	1	g
product (mL)	50	100

By 'spotting':

$$g = 2$$

Therefore, 100 mL of product contains 2 g of ingredient.
 After dilution, the amount of the ingredient remains the same (2 g) and the total amount of the vehicle becomes 1000 mL. Setting up proportional sets for the diluted product:

	amount	percentage	ratio	amount strength (g/mL)
ingredient (g)	2	p	1	a
product (mL)	1000	100	r	1

(*continued*)

By 'spotting':

$p = 0.2$

$r = \left(\dfrac{1000}{2}\right) = 500$

$a = 0.002$

Converting 0.002 g to milligrams:

	g	–	–	mg	
0.002 g =	0	0	0	2	= 2 mg

The final solution can therefore be expressed as a percentage strength of 0.2% w/v, a ratio strength of 1 in 500 w/v or an amount strength of 2 mg/mL.

Serial dilutions

Rather than keeping large amounts of products in the dispensary it is usual to keep concentrated products. These stock solutions can then be diluted to the desired concentration for the final product.

Example 5.3 starts with a ratio strength.

Example 5.3

What volume of a 1 in 400 v/v solution is needed to produce 5 L of a 1 in 2000 v/v solution?

Let y mL be the volume of 1 in 400 solution required.

The amount of the ingredient is the same in both y mL of 1 in 400 solution and 5 L of 1 in 2000 solution. Let this amount be x mL. Setting up proportional sets:

For 1 in 400 v/v:

ingredient (mL)	1	x
product (mL)	400	y

→

For 5 L of 1 in 2000 v/v:

ingredient (mL)   1   x

product (mL)   2000   5000

From the second pair, by 'spotting':

$$x = \frac{5000}{2000} = 2.5$$

Now putting x in the first pair of proportional sets:
For 1 in 400 v/v:

ingredient (mL)   1   2.5

product (mL)   400   y

Therefore:

$$y = 400 \times 2.5 = 1000$$

So 1000 mL or 1 L of the 1 in 400 mixture is diluted to 5 L to produce a 1 in 2000 product.

Example 5.4 starts with a percentage strength.

Example 5.4

What volume of a 40% v/v solution needs to be used to produce 500 mL of 5% v/v solution?

Let y mL equal the volume of the 40% v/v solution required and let x mL equal the volume of ingredient in y mL of 40% v/v solution. There will also be x mL of ingredient in 500 mL of the 5% v/v solution. Setting up proportional sets:

(*continued*)

For 40% v/v:

  ingredient (mL)   40 x

  product (mL)   100 y

For 500 mL of 5% v/v:

  ingredient (mL)   5 x

  product (mL)   100   500

By 'spotting':

  $x = 25$

Putting x in the first pair of proportional sets:
For 40% v/v:

  ingredient (mL)   40   25

  product (mL)   100 y

Setting up and solving equations:

$$\frac{y}{25} = \frac{100}{40}$$

$$y = \frac{100 \times 25}{40}$$

$$y = 62.5$$

Therefore, 62.5 mL of the 40% v/v solution is required to produce 500 mL of 5% v/v solution.

Sometimes we are required to calculate the amount of diluent required to produce a stated final concentration.

Example 5.5

To what volume must 250 mL of a 25% w/v solution be diluted to produce a 10% solution?

$\rightarrow$

First calculate the amount of ingredient in 250 mL of 25% solution.

Let the number of grams of ingredient in 250 mL of 25% w/v solution be x. By convention, 25% w/v solution has 25 g of ingredient in 100 mL of product. Setting up proportional sets:

For 250 mL of a 25% w/v:

ingredient (g)   25 x

product (mL)   100   250

Corresponding pairs are in the same ratio:

$$\frac{25}{100} = \frac{x}{250}$$

Solving for the unknown value:

$$x = \frac{25 \times 250}{100}$$

$$x = 62.5$$

After dilution, the amount of the ingredient will stay the same, i.e. 62.5 g.

Let y mL be the final volume of the 10% w/v solution. Setting up proportional sets:

For 10% w/v:

ingredient (g)   10   62.5

product (mL)   100 y

By 'spotting' it can be seen that:

$$y = 625\,mL$$

We need to dilute 250 mL of a 25% w/v solution to 625 mL to produce a 10% w/v solution.

Concentrated waters

Concentrated waters, such as rose water, peppermint water and chloroform water, are used to produce single-strength products. They are intended for dilution in the ratio 1 part of concentrated water with 39 parts of water. To produce the single-strength product, we take one part of the concentrate and dilute it to 40 parts with water.

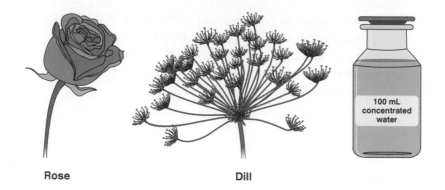

Rose   **Dill**

Suppose that we have to make volumes of single-strength chloroform water (50 mL, 100 mL, 200 mL, 300 mL, 500 mL) from chloroform water concentrate. Since chloroform water concentrate is in the ratio 1 : 40, we have to take 1 mL and dilute it to 40 mL with water in order to obtain single-strength chloroform water.

Setting up proportional sets:

chloroform water concentrate (mL)	1	a	b	c	d	e
water (mL) to		40	50	100	200	300	500

If we calculate the value for c:

$$\frac{1}{40} = \frac{c}{200}$$

$$c = \frac{200}{40} = 5$$

We therefore require 5 mL of chloroform water concentrate made up to 200 mL with water to produce 200 mL of single-strength chloroform water.

This calculation can be repeated for a, b, d and e. Alternatively, these values can be obtained from the value for c by 'spotting', as follows:

$$b = \frac{c}{2} = 2.5$$

$$a = \frac{b}{2} = 1.25$$

$$d = b \times 3 = 7.5$$

$$e = b \times 5 = 12.5$$

Thus, the following proportional sets are obtained for single-strength chloroform water:

chloroform water concentrate (mL)	1	1.25	2.5	5	7.5	12.5
water (mL) to		40	50	100	200	300	500

In most formulae the chloroform water is expressed as double strength for half the total volume. To make double-strength chloroform water we have to take twice the volume of the chloroform water concentrate.

To produce double-strength chloroform water:

chloroform water concentrate (mL)	2	2.5	5	10	15	25
water (mL) to		40	50	100	200	300	500

Simple dilution

Triturations

One of the problems when weighing ingredients for preparations is that amounts of less than 100 mg cannot be weighed with sufficient accuracy. We have to use trituration to get the required amount.

Example 5.6

How would you prepare 100 mL of a preparation to the following formula?

hyoscine hydrobromide (micrograms)	*500*
chloroform water (mL) to	*5*

Let *y* be the number of micrograms of hyoscine hydrobromide in 100 mL. Setting up proportional sets:

hyoscine hydrobromide (micrograms)	500	y
chloroform water (mL) to	5	100

(continued)

By 'spotting':

$y = 10\,000$ micrograms

Converting 10 000 micrograms to milligrams:

	mg	–	–	micrograms	
10 000 micrograms =	1	0	0 0 0		= 10 mg

The problem that we face is that we cannot weigh less than 100 mg with sufficient accuracy.

Let the number of millilitres of product that contains 100 mg of hyoscine hydrobromide be x. Setting up proportional sets:

hyoscine hydrobromide (mg)	10	100
chloroform water (mL) to	100	x

By 'spotting':

$x = 1000$

If we can only weigh 100 mg of hyoscine hydrobromide we would have to make this up to 1000 mL with chloroform water to get the required strength.

Alternative method

We could dissolve 100 mg of hyoscine hydrobromide in a known quantity of chloroform water (say 10 mL) and take out a volume of chloroform water that contained 10 mg of hyoscine hydrobromide and dilute this to 100 mL.

Let us weigh 100 mg of hyoscine hydrobromide and make up to 10 mL with chloroform water. We now need to know the number of millilitres of product that contain 10 mg of hyoscine hydrobromide. Let this be z. Setting up proportional sets:

hyoscine hydrobromide (mg)	100	10
chloroform water (mL) to	10	z

$\rightarrow$

By 'spotting':

$z = 1$

If we take 1 mL of this solution we have 10 mg of hyoscine hydrobromide. We can then dilute this to 100 mL with chloroform water to get the required solution.

In the original method we used up to 1000 mL of chloroform water but in the alternative method only 110 mL was used.

If we had chosen to dissolve the 100 mg of hyoscine hydrobromide in 100 mL of chloroform water, we would proceed as follows.

Let a be the number of millilitres of product containing 10 mg of hyoscine hydrobromide. Setting up proportional sets:

hyoscine hydrobromide (mg)	100	10
chloroform water (mL) to	100	a

By 'spotting':

$a = 10$

We would make 10 mL of this solution up to 100 mL with chloroform water. In this situation we would use 200 mL of chloroform water overall.

The aim should be to dissolve the hyoscine hydrobromide to produce the required amount of solution with the least wastage. The solubility of the ingredient needs to be considered.

Powder calculations

The Pharmaceutical Codex states that powders must weigh a minimum of 120 mg. No maximum weight is stated. If the amount of drug in the powder is less than 120 mg, it is necessary to include an inert powder to bulk up the powder to the minimum weight.

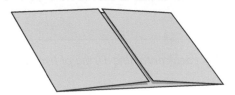

Example 5.7

Prepare five powders each containing 100 mg of paracetamol.
Setting up proportional sets for one and five powders:

number of powders	1	5
paracetamol (mg)	100	*a*
diluent (mg)	*y*	*b*
total weight (mg)	120	*c*

y is the amount of diluent required to increase the final weight of one powder to 120 mg, therefore:

$$y = 120 - 100 = 20$$

a is the amount of paracetamol in five powders, *b* is the amount of diluent and *c* is the total weight of the five powders. The ratio of the powders is 1 to 5 so we can calculate these values by multiplying by 5:

number of powders	1	5
paracetamol (mg)	100	500
diluent (mg)	20	100
total weight (mg)	120	600

To prepare five powders each containing 100 mg of paracetamol, we need to weigh 500 mg of paracetamol and add it to 100 mg of diluent. This mixture would then be divided into five powders of 120 mg.

In Example 5.8 powders containing a smaller quantity of drug are considered.

Example 5.8

Prepare five powders each containing 10 mg of hyoscine hydrobromide.

→

Setting up proportional sets for one and five powders:

number of powders	1	5
hyoscine hydrobromide(mg)	10	a
diluent (mg)	y	b
total weight (mg)	120	c

Therefore:

$$y = 120 - 10 = 110$$

number of powders	1	5
hyoscine hydrobromide (mg)	10	50
diluent (mg)	110	550
total weight (mg)	120	600

As has been stated before we cannot accurately weigh less than 100 mg, so we have two alternatives: either make up the powders with 100 mg hyoscine hydrobromide or triturate the powders.

If we make up the powders with 100 mg of hyoscine hydrobromide we get:

number of powders	1	g
hyoscine hydrobromide (mg)	10	100
diluent (mg)	110	e
total weight (mg)	120	f

We can see that the hyoscine hydrobromide is in the ratio 1 to 10, so g, e and f are 10, 1100 and 1200, respectively, and we have therefore made enough for 10 powders.

Alternatively, we can use the trituration method. We take 100 mg of hyoscine hydrobromide and dilute it with 900 mg of diluent. We need to know what weight of powder contains 50 mg of hyoscine hydrobromide. Let that be n. Setting up proportional sets:

hyoscine hydrobromide (mg)	100	50
diluent (mg)	900	m
powder (mg)	1000	n

(continued)

By 'spotting':

$n = 500$

We can therefore take 500 mg of this mixture and subtract that from the weight of five powders of 120 mg each:

$5 \times 120 = 600\,mg$

Subtracting:

$600 - 500 = 100\,mg$

If we take 500 mg of the triturate and add another 100 mg of diluent we have enough to make five powders each weighing 120 mg and containing 10 mg of hyoscine hydrobromide.

To prepare five powders of 10 mg hyoscine hydrobromide, we weigh 100 mg of hyoscine hydrobromide and add 900 mg of diluent. We then take 500 mg of this mixture and add 100 mg of diluent. The final mixture is then divided into five powders of 120 mg.

Example 5.9 shows how additional triturations can be used to achieve the required dose in the final product.

Example 5.9

Prepare six powders each containing 0.5 mg of drug.

Setting up proportional sets for one and six powders:

number of powders	1	6
drug (mg)	0.5	a
diluent (mg)	Y	b
total weight (mg)	120	c

$\rightarrow$

Therefore:

$$y = 120 - 0.5 = 119.5$$

The figures are in the ratio of 1 to 6 so the proportional sets become:

number of powders	1	6
drug (mg)	0.5	3
diluent (mg)	119.5	717
total weight (mg)	120	720

Again we cannot weigh less than 100 mg of drug.

Let z equal the number of powders containing a total of 100 mg of drug:

number of powders	1	z
drug (mg)	0.5	100
diluent (mg)	119.5	d
total weight (mg)	120	e

By 'spotting':

$$z = 200$$

Giving values for d and e:

number of powders	1	200
drug (mg)	0.5	100
diluent (mg)	119.5	23 900
total weight (mg)	120	24 000

We would have to make enough for 200 powders and try to mix 100 mg of drug with 23 900 mg of diluent.

Alternatively, we could use trituration. Weigh 100 mg of drug and mix with 900 mg and call this T1.

(continued)

Let the weight of powder containing 3 mg of drug (i.e. sufficient for six powders) be y:

T1

drug (mg)	100	3
total weight (mg)	1000	y

By 'spotting'

$$y = 30$$

Therefore, 30 mg of powder contains 3 mg of drug.

We still cannot weigh this amount of powder, so we need to take 100 mg of T1 (which is one-tenth of the total product of T1 and will contain 10 mg of drug) and add 900 mg of diluent to produce T2.

Let the weight of T2 containing 3 mg of drug be z:

T2

drug (mg)	10	3
total weight (mg)	1000	z

In this case $z = 300$, so 300 mg of T2 contains 3 mg of drug and we can weigh 300 mg.

The final weight for six powders is:

$$6 \times 120 = 720 \text{ mg}$$

We therefore take 300 mg of T2 and subtract:

$$720 - 300 = 420 \text{ mg of diluent}$$

By using this method we are creating different concentrations of mixtures:

T1 contains 100 mg of drug in 1000 mg of powder = 1 mg in 10 mg

T2 contains 10 mg of drug in 1000 mg of powder = 1 mg in 100 mg

T3 contains 1 mg of drug in 1000 mg of powder = 1 mg in 1000 mg and so on.

Multiple dilutions

We now consider how to calculate the amount of ingredient required in the initial product when given the final concentration and the degree of dilution.

Example 5.10

What weight of ingredient is required to produce 1000 mL of a solution such that, when 2.5 mL of it is diluted to 50 mL with water, it gives a 0.25% w/v solution?

Consider the 0.25% w/v solution and let y g be the weight of ingredient in 100 mL. By convention, 0.25% w/v means 0.25 g in 100 mL.
For 100 mL of 0.25% w/v:

    ingredient (g)   0.25 y

    water (mL) to   100   50

We can see that $y = 0.125$.
    Now we take 2.5 mL of the original solution and increase the volume to 50 mL. The amount of ingredient will stay the same, i.e. y, so we get proportional sets that relate the weight of ingredient in 50 mL to the weight in 2.5 mL.
    Let z be the number of grams of ingredient in 1000 mL of solution:

    ingredient (g) z y

    water (mL) to   1000   2.5

We know that $y = 0.125$, so:

    ingredient (g) z 0.125

    water (mL) to   1000   2.5

By 'spotting':

    $z = 50$

Therefore, the original solution is 50 g of ingredient made up to 1000 mL with water.

Example 5.11

What weight of malachite green oxalate is required to produce 500 mL of solution such that 25 mL of this solution diluted to 4000 L gives a 1 in 2 000 000 solution?

Start by converting the litres into millilitres so that all the units are the same:

$$L \quad - \quad - \quad mL$$

$$4000\,L= \quad 4 \quad 0 \quad 0 \quad 0 \quad 0 \quad 0 \quad 0 \quad =4\,000\,000\,mL$$

Let the amount of malachite green oxalate in 4 000 000 mL be y. Setting up proportional sets:

malachite green oxalate(g)	1	y
water (mL) to	2 000 000	4 000 000

By 'spotting':

$$y = 2$$

As we took 25 mL of the original and diluted it to 4 000 000 mL, we know that 25 mL contains 2 g of malachite green oxalate because we have only increased the volume and the amount has stayed the same.

Let z be the amount of malachite green oxalate in the 500 mL of original solution. Setting up proportional sets:

malachite green oxalate (g)	z	2
water (mL) to	500	25

Corresponding values are in the same ratio:

$$\frac{z}{500} = \frac{2}{25}$$

Solving the equation for the unknown:

$$z = \frac{2 \times 500}{25} = 40$$

Therefore, 40 g of malachite green oxalate is dissolved in water to produce 500 mL of solution.

Example 5.12

What weight of ingredient is required to produce 250 mL of a solution such that 10 mL of this solution diluted to 150 mL gives a 0.1% w/v solution?

Let z be the number of grams of ingredient in 250 mL of unknown strength product and y be the number of grams of ingredient in 10 mL of unknown strength product. The amount of ingredient in the final 150 mL of 0.1% solution will also be y. Setting up proportional sets:

for the unknown strength product:

ingredient (g)	z	y
product (mL)	250	10

for the final solution of 0.1% w/v:

ingredient (g)	y	0.1
product (mL)	150	100

Corresponding values are in the same ratio:

$$\frac{y}{150} = \frac{0.1}{100}$$

Solving the equation for the unknown:

$$y = \frac{150 \times 0.1}{100}$$

$$y = 0.15$$

Putting this value into the first pair of proportional sets:

ingredient (g)	z	0.15
product (mL)	250	10

Corresponding values are in the same ratio:

$$\frac{z}{250} = \frac{0.15}{10}$$

$$z = \frac{0.15 \times 250}{10} = 3.75$$

Therefore, we take 3.75 g of ingredient and make it up to 250 mL with water.

Examples 5.13 and 5.14 demonstrate how to calculate the amount of initial product of stated strength that is required to produce a stated volume of a final strength.

Example 5.13

How many millilitres of 0.5% w/v solution are required to produce 250 mL of 1 in 5000 solution?

By convention, 0.5% w/v means 0.5 g in 100 mL.

Let the number of millilitres of 0.5% solution be y and the number of grams of ingredient in 250 mL of a 1 in 5000 solution be x. The amount of ingredient in grams in y mL of 0.5% solution will also be x. Setting up proportional sets:

for 0.5% w/v:

ingredient (g)	0.5	x
product (mL)	100	y

for 250 mL of 1 in 5000:

ingredient (g)	1	x
product (mL)	5000	250

Corresponding pairs are in the same ratio:

$$\frac{1}{5000} = \frac{x}{250}$$

Solving for the unknown:

$$x = \frac{250}{5000}$$

$$x = 0.05$$

Substituting into the first pair of proportional sets:

for 0.5% w/v:

ingredient (g)	0.5	0.05
product (mL)	100	y

→

By 'spotting':

$y = 10$

Therefore, 10 mL of 0.5% solution will produce 250 mL of 1 in 5000 solution.

Example 5.14

How many millilitres of a 1 in 80 w/v solution are required to make 500 mL of a 0.02% solution?

By convention, 1 in 80 means 1 g in 80 mL and 0.02% w/v means 0.02 g in 100 mL.
  Let the number of millilitres of the 1 in 80 solution be *y* and let the amount of ingredient in grams in 500 mL of 0.02% solution be *x*. The amount of ingredient in grams in *y* mL of 1 in 80 solution will also be *x*. Setting up proportional sets:

for 1 in 80:

ingredient (g)	1	*x*
product (mL)	80	*y*

for 500 mL of 0.02%:

ingredient (g)	0.02	*x*
product (mL)	100	500

By 'spotting':

$x = 0.1$

Substituting into the first pair of proportional sets:

for 1 in 80:

ingredient (g)	1	0.1
product (mL)	80	*y*

(continued)

By 'spotting':

$y = 8$

Therefore, 8 mL of a 1 in 80 w/v solution is required to make 500 mL of a 0.02% w/v solution.

Mixing concentrations

There are situations when two or more strengths of product are mixed at stated volumes and the final concentration must be calculated.

Example 5.15

What is the final % v/v of a solution if 200 mL of 40% v/v solution is added to 300 mL of 70% v/v solution?

The two volumes will be added together to make the final volume of 500 mL. The volumes of ingredients present in the two volumes will therefore need to be added together.

Let x mL be the volume of ingredient in 200 mL of 40% v/v solution. Setting up proportional sets:

ingredient (mL)	40	x
product (mL)	100	200

By 'spotting':

$x = 80$

Let y be the number of millilitres of ingredient in 300 mL of 70% v/v solution. Setting up proportional sets:

ingredient (mL)	70	y
product (mL)	100	300

By 'spotting':

$y = 210$

$\rightarrow$

The total volume of ingredient in 500 mL of final solution is:

$80 + 210 = 290$ mL

Let p be the percentage strength. Setting up proportional sets:

ingredient (mL)   290 p

product (mL)   500   100

By 'spotting':

$p = 58$

Therefore, the final solution is 58% v/v.

Sometimes we are required to calculate the ratio in which two different products of given strengths must be mixed to produce a product of a given concentration.

Let us consider what happens when two products of different concentrations are mixed. The final volume is the sum of the two volumes and the final amount is the sum of the two amounts present in the volumes used.

For product 1 let the concentration be c_1, the volume of product used be v_1 and the amount of ingredient in v_1 be a_1. These values are c_2, v_2 and a_2 for product 2 and c_3, v_3 and a_3 for the final combined product.

The volume of product 1 (v_1) + volume of product 2 (v_2) = volume of final product (v_3), i.e.

$v_1 + v_2 = v_3$

The amount of ingredient in v_1 (a_1) + amount of ingredient in v_2 (a_2) = amount of ingredient in v_3 (a_3), i.e.

$a_1 + a_2 = a_3$

If c_1 is the concentration of product 1 (expressed as a fraction or a decimal):

$$c_1 = \frac{a_1}{v_1}$$

$a_1 = v_1 c_1$

$a_1 + a_2 = a_3$

$$(v_1 \times c_1) + (v_2 \times c_2) = (v_3 \times c_3)$$

$$(v_1 \times c_1) + (v_2 \times c_2) = (v_1 + v_2) \times c_3$$

$$(v_1 \times c_1) + (v_2 \times c_2) = (v_1 \times v_3) + (v_2 \times c_3)$$

$$(v_1 \times c_1) - (v_1 \times c_3) = (v_2 \times c_3) - (v_2 \times c_2)$$

$$v_1 \times (c_1 - c_3) = v_2 \times (c_3 - c_2)$$

therefore:

$$\frac{v_1}{v_2} = \frac{(c_3 - c_2)}{(c_1 - c_3)}$$

In some textbooks this has been shown graphically as follows:

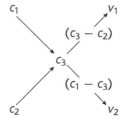

Example 5.16

A suspension used to be provided as two strengths, both 100 mg/5 mL and 25 mg/5 mL solutions, which could be mixed to produce intermediate doses. If we want to produce a product that has a strength of 75 mg/5 mL, what proportion of the two mixtures do we need?

$$c_1 = \frac{100\ mg}{5\ mL} = 20$$

$$c_2 = \frac{25\ mg}{5\ mL} = 5$$

$$c_3 = \frac{75\ mg}{5\ mL} = 15$$

$$\frac{v_1}{v_2} = \frac{(15 - 5)}{(20 - 15)} = \frac{10}{5} = \frac{2}{1}$$

→

or graphically:

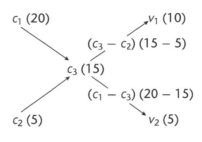

We therefore need 2 parts 100 mg/5 mL solution and 1 part 25 mg/5 mL solution to produce a 75 mg/5 mL solution.

We can show that this works if we are required to make 300 mL of 75 mg/5 mL suspension. Using the above proportions we add 2 parts of suspension containing 100 mg/5 mL solution, i.e. 200 mL (v_1) and 1 part of the 25 mg/5 mL suspension, i.e. 100 mL (v_2).

Let a_1 be the amount of drug in milligrams in 200 mL of 100 mg/5 mL suspension. Setting up proportional sets:

drug (mg)   100 a_1

product (mL)   5   200

By 'spotting':

$a_1 = 4000$

Let y be the number of milligrams of drug in 100 mL of 25 mg/5 mL suspension. Setting up proportional sets:

Drug (mg)   25 a_2

product (mL)   5   100

By 'spotting':

$a_2 = 500$

The amount of drug in 300 mL of final product is a_3:

$a_1 + a_2 = a_3 = 4500$

(*continued*)

Let the final strength be y mg in 5 mL. Setting up proportional sets:

drug (mg)   4500 y

product (mL)   300   5

Corresponding values are in the same ratio:

$$\frac{4500}{300} = \frac{y}{5}$$

Solving for the unknown:

$$y = \frac{4500 \times 5}{300}$$

$$y = 75$$

Therefore, the solution is 75 mg/5 mL, as expected.

Example 5.17

Find the proportions of the same two suspensions given in Example 5.16 that would be required to produce a 50 mg/5 mL suspension.

$c_1 = 20$

$c_2 = 5$

$c_3 = 10$

$$\frac{v_1}{v_2} = \frac{(10 - 5)}{(20 - 10)} = \frac{5}{10} = \frac{1}{2}$$

Graphically:

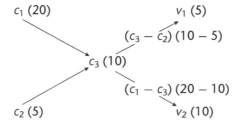

c_1 (20) v_1 (5)

$(c_3 - c_2)$ (10 − 5)

c_3 (10)

$(c_1 - c_3)$ (20 − 10)

c_2 (5) v_2 (10)

$\rightarrow$

Therefore: $\dfrac{v_1}{v_2} = \dfrac{5}{10} = \dfrac{1}{2}.$

We therefore mix 1 part 100 mg/5 mL solution with 2 parts 25 mg/5 mL solution.

Example 5.18

What proportions of 90% v/v and 50% v/v ethanol mixtures would produce a 70% v/v mixture? Assume no contraction.

$$c_1 = \frac{90}{100} = 0.9$$

$$c_2 = \frac{50}{100} = 0.5$$

$$c_3 = \frac{70}{100} = 0.7$$

Provided that all the terms have the same denominator this division can be omitted.

$$\frac{v_1}{v_2} = \frac{(0.7 - 0.5)}{(0.9 - 0.7)} = \frac{0.2}{0.2} = \frac{1}{1}$$

Graphically

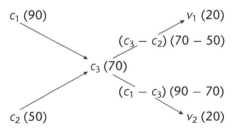

c_1 (90) v_1 (20)

                          $(c_3 - c_2)$ (70 − 50)

                  c_3 (70)

                          $(c_1 - c_3)$ (90 − 70)

c_2 (50) v_2 (20)

(continued)

We therefore need to mix 1 part 90% solution with 1 part 50% solution.
    We can prove this is correct. If we mix 100 mL of 90% solution and 100 mL of 50% solution we expect the final strength to be 70%.
    Let a_1 be the number of millilitres of ethanol in 100 mL of 90% solution. Setting up proportional sets:

ethanol (mL)   90 a_1

product (mL)   100   100

By 'spotting':

$a_1 = 90$

Let a_2 be the number of millilitres of ethanol in 100 mL of 50% solution. Setting up proportional sets:

ethanol (mL)   50 a_2

product (mL)   100   100

By 'spotting':

$a_2 = 50$

Therefore, the final product contains an ethanol volume of a_3 in 200 mL.

$a_3 = a_1 + a_2 = 50 + 90 = 140$

Let p be the percentage strength of the final product. Setting up proportional sets:

ethanol (mL)   140 p

product (mL)   200   100

By 'spotting':

$p = 70$

Therefore, the final product is 70% v/v and the ratio is correct.

Mixing two concentrations without a final volume

Answers are given at the end of the chapter.

Q1   What weight of potassium permanganate is required to produce 300 mL of solution such that 5 mL of this solution diluted to 250 mL gives a 0.01% w/v solution?

Q2   What weight of potassium permanganate is required to produce 500 mL of solution such that 25 mL of this solution diluted to 500 mL gives a 0.025% w/v solution?

Q3   What weight of zinc sulfate is required to produce 150 mL of solution such that 10 mL of this solution diluted to 200 mL gives a 1% w/v solution?

Q4   What weight of potassium permanganate is required to produce 200 mL of solution such that 50 mL of this solution diluted to 200 mL will produce a 1 in 400 solution?

Q5   What weight of malachite green oxalate is required to produce 300 mL of a solution such that 25 mL of this solution diluted to 2000 L gives a 0.5 ppm solution?

Q6   How many millilitres of water must be added to 180 mL of 40% v/v solution in order to produce a 5% v/v solution?

Q7   What weight of copper sulfate is required to produce 150 mL of solution such that 30 mL of this solution diluted to 150 mL produces a 1 in 6000 solution?

Q8   What weight of potassium permanganate is needed to produce 300 mL of solution such that if 1 mL is diluted to 20 mL a 0.1% w/v solution is produced?

Q9   What volume of 100 mg/5 mL solution is required to be diluted to give 200 mL of 75 mg/5 mL solution?

Q10   How many millilitres of 90% alcohol when diluted to 135 mL produces 60% alcohol? (Assume no contraction in volume.)

Q11 When 70 mL of sodium chloride 0.9% w/v solution is combined with 100 mL of 1.7% w/v sodium chloride solution what is the final strength of the solution?

Q12 What volume of a 0.6% w/v solution is required to produce 200 mL of 1 in 10 000 solution?

Q13 What volume of a 1 in 50 solution is required to produce 300 mL of a 0.3% w/v solution?

Q14 Calculate the volumes of two stock solutions of 100 mg/5 mL and 25 mg/5 mL that must be mixed to produce 500 mL of 75 mg/5 mL solution.

Q15 What volumes of two stock solutions of 30% w/v and 60% w/v are required to make 300 mL of 40% w/v solution?

Q16 Calculate the volume of 0.2% w/v potassium permanganate solution required to produce 1000 mL of a 100 ppm solution.

Answers

A1 1.5 g

A2 2.5 g

A3 30 g

A4 2 g

A5 12 g

A6 1260 mL

A7 125 mg

A8 6 g

A9 150 mL

A10 90 mL

A11 1.37%

A12 3.3 mL

A13 45 mL

A14 167 mL of 25 mg/5 mL solution and 333 mL of 100 mg/5 mL solution

A15 100 mL of 60% solution and 200 mL of 30% solution

A16 50 mL

6

Formulations

Learning objectives

By the end of this chapter you will be able to:

- manipulate a given formula to the amount required on the prescription
- check the calculated amounts against the original formula to ensure accuracy
- state the difference between the terms 'parts' and 'to parts'

Formulae in pharmacy are recipes from either the standard literature available or the directions of the prescriber. Ingredients can be listed as amounts, parts or percentages. The formula may also have the amount in a greater or smaller quantity than is written on the prescription.

Formulae in pharmacy originate from a period of time when all preparations were made specifically for an individual patient. At that time pharmaceutical companies did not exist. As a pharmacy student you are likely to have used these formulae when preparing preparations extemporaneously. These preparations may contain several active and inactive ingredients and so there are several calculations to complete. An error in any of these calculations has the potential to cause harm to the patient.

As ingredients with a formula have to be kept in fixed ratios, they form proportional sets. Comparison of numbers in the sets after calculation, to ensure that the proportions are maintained, is a valuable way of checking the formula and should overcome the potential for error.

Using proportional sets provides a structured approach to the problem and provides you with a method for checking accuracy.

Reducing the formula

Some reference sources provide a formula for a larger quantity than the quantity required on the prescription.

Example 6.1

A prescription requires 200 mL of Chalk Mixture, Paediatric BP. The formula is:

chalk	20 g
tragacanth powder	2 g
cinnamon water, concentrated	4 mL
syrup	100 mL
chloroform water, double strength	500 mL
water for preparation to	1000 mL

We therefore have a formula to produce 1000 mL of the preparation but require 200 mL. Calculate the quantities required to produce 200 mL.

Setting up proportional sets:

	master formula	to make 200 mL
chalk (g)	20	a
tragacanth powder (g)	2	b
cinnamon water, concentrated (mL)	4	c
syrup (mL)	100	d
chloroform water, double strength (mL)	500	e
water for preparation (mL) to	1000	200

We can calculate the missing values by setting up the ratio equations for corresponding pairs or by spotting.
To calculate the amount of chalk we pick out the proportional sets:

chalk (g)	20	a
water for preparation (mL) to	1000	200

By 'spotting', 1000 is divided by 5 to get 200, so 20 is divided by 5 to get:

$a = 4$

→

Continuing the process for other pairs of ingredients we get:

	master formula	to make 200 mL
chalk (g)	20	4
tragacanth powder (g)	2	0.4
cinnamon water, concentrated (mL)	4	0.8
syrup (mL)	100	20
chloroform water, double strength (mL)	500	100
water for preparation (mL) to	1000	200

At this stage it is important to check the relative amounts of the ingredients and re-check the ratios in order to eliminate any errors.

Increasing the formula

Some reference sources provide a formula that is for a smaller quantity than the quantity required on the prescription.

Example 6.2

Calculate the quantities required to produce 300 mL of Aromatic Magnesium Carbonate Mixture BP using the formula:

light magnesium carbonate	300 mg
sodium bicarbonate	500 mg
aromatic cardamom tincture	0.3 mL
chloroform water, double strength	5 mL
water to	10 mL

(continued)

Setting up proportional sets:

	master formula	to make 300 mL
light magnesium carbonate (mg)	300	a
sodium bicarbonate (mg)	500	b
aromatic cardamom tincture (mL)	0.3	c
chloroform water, double strength (mL)	5	d
water (mL) to	10	300

Picking out two proportional sets:

light magnesium carbonate (mg)	300	a
water (mL) to	10	300

Corresponding pairs are in the same ratio so:

$$\frac{300}{10} = \frac{a}{300}$$

Solving for the unknown:

$$a = \frac{300 \times 300}{10}$$

$$a = 9000$$

We continue the process to get:

	master formula	to make 300 mL
light magnesium carbonate (mg)	300	9000
sodium bicarbonate (mg)	500	15 000
aromatic cardamom tincture (mL)	0.3	9
chloroform water, double strength (mL)	5	150
water (mL) to	10	300

Again, a thorough check of the corresponding values should be made.

Formulae involving parts

Sometimes the formula for a product is expressed as parts rather than as quantities. The total amount of product will be the sum of the parts of the ingredients. From this, a formula can be produced and used to calculate the amounts of the ingredients in a required amount of product.

Example 6.3

Consider the standard for Industrial Methylated Spirit (IMS) BP, which states that ingredients should be in the ratio 95 parts spirit to 5 parts wood naphtha. (In the BNF this is stated as 19 volumes of ethanol and 1 volume of approved wood naphtha, which is the same). In IMS both the ingredients are liquids so the parts are volume in volume. How much of each ingredient is required to produce 300 L?

Setting up proportional sets:

	master formula	to make 300 L
spirit (L)	95	a
wood naphtha (L)	5	b
IMS (L)	100 (95 + 5)	300

We can spot that:

$$b = 5 \times 3 = 15$$
$$a = 95 \times 3 = 285$$

Therefore, the proportional sets become:

	master formula	to make 300 L
spirit (L)	95	285
wood naphtha (L)	5	15
IMS (L)	100	300

Example 6.4 involves solids in a formula expressed as parts.

Example 6.4

Find the quantities of ingredients needed to produce 50 g of product using the formula:

calamine (parts weight)	*2*
yellow soft paraffin (parts weight)	*38*

The total ointment contains 40 parts $(2 + 38)$. Setting up the proportional sets:

	master formula	to produce 50 g
calamine (g)	2	x
yellow soft paraffin (g)	38	y
total (g)	40	50

Corresponding pairs of values are in the same ratio:

$$\frac{2}{40} = \frac{x}{50}$$

Solving for the unknown:

$$x = \frac{2 \times 50}{40}$$

$$x = 2.5$$

Therefore:

$$y = 50 - 2.5 = 47.5$$

The proportional sets become:

	master formula	to produce 50 g
calamine (g)	2	2.5
yellow soft paraffin (g)	38	47.5
total (g)	40	50

It is necessary to differentiate carefully between the use of 'parts' and 'to parts'. Compare the following two formulae:

Formula 1

| calamine | 1 part |
| white soft paraffin | 10 parts |

This is equivalent to:

| calamine | 1 g |
| white soft paraffin | 10 g |

This is a total of 11 g (or 11 parts).

Formula 2

| calamine | 1 part |
| white soft paraffin to | 10 parts |

This is equivalent to:

| calamine | 1 g |
| white soft paraffin | 9 g |

This is a total of 10 g (or 10 parts).

Formulae containing percentages

A formula can also be expressed in percentages. Ointments and creams are the most common examples of this. The percentages of the ingredients can be used to produce the formula and the ingredients in a known amount of product can be calculated.

Example 6.5

Using the following formula, calculate the amounts of ingredients required to make 25 g:

sulfur	*6%*
salicylic acid	*4%*
white soft paraffin to	*100%*

Setting up proportional sets:

	master formula	to make 25 g
sulfur (g)	6	*a*
salicylic acid (g)	4	*b*
white soft paraffin (g)	90	*c*
total ointment (g)	100	25

100 is divided by 4 to get 25, therefore, by 'spotting', each amount in the first column is divided by 4 to get the corresponding amount in the second column. The result is:

	master formula	to make 25 g
sulfur (g)	6	1.5
salicylic acid (g)	4	1
white soft paraffin (g)	90	22.5
total ointment (g)	100	25

Example 6.6

Find the amount of ingredients required to make 50 g of the following formulation:

calamine	*6% w/w*
liquid paraffin	*7% w/w*
yellow soft paraffin to	*100% w/w*

→

Setting up proportional sets:

	master formula	to make 50 g
calamine (g)	6	a
liquid paraffin (g)	7	b
yellow soft paraffin (g)	87	c
total product	100	50

By 'spotting':

$a = 3$

$b = 3.5$

$c = 43.5$

The formula is therefore:

	master formula	to make 50 g
calamine (g)	6	3
liquid paraffin (g)	7	3.5
yellow soft paraffin (g)	87	43.5

Practice calculations

Answers are given at the end of the chapter.

Q1   Calculate the amounts of the following required to produce 200 g of cream:

calamine	10%
zinc oxide	15%
aqueous cream to	100%

Q2   Calculate the formula for 20 g of benzoic acid ointment compound using the formula:

benzoic acid	6%
salicylic acid	4%
emulsifying ointment to	100%

Q3   Calculate the formula required to produce 300 mL of menthol and eucalyptus inhalation from the formula:

menthol	2 g
eucalyptus oil	10 g
light magnesium carbonate	7 g
water to	100 mL

Q4   Calculate the amounts of ingredients required to make 30 g of ointment to the following formula:

coal tar solution	12% w/w
hydrous wool fat	24% w/w
yellow soft paraffin to	100%

Q5   Calamine and Coal Tar Ointment BP has the following formula:

calamine	12.5 g
strong coal tar solution	2.5 g
zinc oxide	12.5 g
hydrous wool fat	25 g
white soft paraffin	47.5 g

Calculate the amounts of ingredients required to produce 25 g of product.

Q6   Zinc and coal tar paste has the following formula:

zinc oxide	6% w/w
coal tar	6% w/w
emulsifying wax	5% w/w
starch	38% w/w
yellow soft paraffin	45% w/w

Calculate the amounts of ingredients required to produce 300 g of paste.

Q7   Calculate the amounts of ingredients required to produce 300 mL of Ammonia and Ipecacuanha Mixture BP, which has the formula:

ammonium bicarbonate	200 mg
liquorice liquid extract	0.5 mL
ipecacuanha tincture	0.3 mL
concentrated camphor water	0.1 mL
concentrated anise water	0.05 mL
double-strength chloroform water	5 mL
water to	10 mL

Q8   Calculate the amounts of ingredients required to make 150 mL of Diamorphine Linctus BPC 1973, which has the formula:

diamorphine hydrochloride	3 mg
oxymel	1.25 mL
glycerol	1.25 mL
compound tartrazine solution	0.06 mL
syrup to	5 mL

Q9   Calculate the amounts of ingredients required to make 3 L of the formula:

witch hazel   4 parts

glycerol   1 part

water   15 parts

Q10   Calculate the amounts of ingredients required to make 2 L of the formula:

aluminium hydroxide   200 mg

simeticone   25 mg

magnesium hydroxide   200 mg

water to   5 mL

Q11   Calculate the amounts of ingredients required to make 30 g of coal tar and zinc ointment using the formula:

strong coal tar solution   100 g

zinc oxide, finely sifted   300 g

yellow soft paraffin   600 g

Q12   Calculate the amounts of ingredients needed to produce 200 mL of kaolin and morphine mixture using the formula:

light kaolin   200 g

sodium bicarbonate   50 g

chloroform and morphine tincture   40 mL

water sufficient to produce   1000 mL

Q13   Calculate using the following formula the amounts of ingredients needed to produce 500 g of product:

calcium carbonate   5 parts

sodium bicarbonate   5 parts

bismuth subcarbonate   3 parts

Q14 Calculate the amounts of ingredients required to make 200 g of product from the formula:

Betnovate ointment   1 part

yellow soft paraffin to   5 parts

Q15 Calculate the amounts of ingredients required to make 300 g of product from the formula:

Betnovate ointment   3 parts

yellow soft paraffin   8 parts

Answers

A1 calamine   20 g
        zinc oxide   30 g
        aqueous cream   150 g

A2 benzoic acid   1.2 g
        salicylic acid   0.8 g
        emulsifying ointment   18 g

A3 menthol   6 g
        eucalyptus oil   30 g
        light magnesium carbonate   21 g
        water to   300 mL

A4 coal tar solution   3.6 g
        hydrous wool fat   7.2 g
        yellow soft paraffin   19.2 g

A5 calamine   3.125 g
        strong coal tar solution   0.625 g
        zinc oxide   3.125 g
        hydrous wool fat   6.25 g
        white soft paraffin   11.875 g

A6 zinc oxide   18 g
        coal tar   18 g
        emulsifying wax   15 g
        starch   114 g
        yellow soft paraffin   135 g

A7 ammonium bicarbonate   6000 mg
        liquorice liquid extract   15 mL
        ipecacuanha tincture   9 mL
        concentrated camphor water   3 mL
        concentrated anise water   1.5 mL
        double-strength chloroform water   150 mL
        water to   300 mL

A8 diamorphine hydrochloride   90 mg
        oxymel   37.5 mL
        glycerol   37.5 mL
        compound tartrazine solution   1.8 mL
        syrup to   150 mL

A9 witch hazel   0.6 L
        glycerol   0.15 L
        water   2.25 L

A10 aluminium hydroxide   80 000 mg
        simeticone   10 000 mg
        magnesium hydroxide   80 000 mg
        water to   2000 mL

A11 strong coal tar solution   3 g
        zinc oxide, finely sifted   9 g
        yellow soft paraffin   18 g

A12 light kaolin   40 g

sodium bicarbonate   10 g

chloroform and morphine tincture   8 mL

water sufficient to produce   200 mL

A13 calcium carbonate   192.3 g

sodium bicarbonate   192.3 g

bismuth subcarbonate   115.4 g

A14 Betnovate ointment   40 g

yellow soft paraffin   160 g

A15 Betnovate ointment   81.8 g

yellow soft paraffin   218.2 g

7

Calculation of doses

Learning objectives

By the end of this chapter you will be able to:

- define the terms 'dose' and 'dosage regimen'
- calculate the total amount of medication required for an individual and to fill a prescription
- convert doses to different dosage forms
- calculate the dose for a patient using weight

To perform calculations involving doses, it is essential to understand the terms 'dose' and 'dosage regimen'.

Dose

A dose is the quantity or amount of a drug or drug formulation taken by, or administered to, a patient to achieve a therapeutic outcome.

The term 'dose' can be further qualified as a single dose, a daily dose, a daily divided dose, a weekly dose, as described with examples below:

- **Single dose**: for example, for self administration in and for treatment of acute anaphylaxis, the *British National Formulary* (BNF)-recommended dose for adrenaline is 300 micrograms, i.e. a single dose of 300 micrograms
- **Daily dose**: for example, the BNF-recommended dose of atorvastatin is 10 mg once daily
- **Daily divided dose**: the recommended initial dose for sodium valproate is 600 mg daily in one or two divided doses, i.e. the dose could be given as one 600 mg dose or the 600 mg dose is divided into two doses of 300 mg each
- **Weekly dose**: mefloquine, when used as an antimalarial, has an adult dosage regimen of 250 mg once weekly.

The dose of a drug may be repeated. For example, in the case of mebendazole for the treatment of threadworm, the BNF states: 'if re-infection [with threadworm] occurs a second dose may be needed after 2 weeks'.

Doses can also be calculated depending on the age, weight or body surface area of the patient. This is particularly true when reviewing the prescribing for children, and will be covered in Chapter 8.

Dosage regimen

A dose may be repeated regularly either throughout the day or following some other time period. Such scheduling of doses is called the dosage regimen.

Examples of different dosage regimens are:

- in the treatment of whipworm, the BNF-recommended dosage of mebendazole is 100 mg twice daily for 3 days, i.e. the dose is 100 mg of mebendazole and the dosage regimen is twice daily for 3 days
- erythromycin has a dosage regimen of 250–500 mg to be taken orally every 6 hours
- clarithromycin has a dosage regimen of 250 mg every 12 hours for 7 days.

Thus doses and dosage regimens vary with the drug and the disease/illness/symptoms that the drug is intended to treat. The dose and dosage regimen of a drug can be found in official publications, such as the BNF and in manufacturers' literature.

Formulations

In addition, a drug may be presented in more than one formulation and in more than one strength. For example, the drug amoxicillin is available in the following formulations:

capsules: 250 mg and 500 mg

suspension: 125 mg/1.25 mL, 125 mg/5 mL, 250 mg/5 mL

sachets: 3 g/sachet

injection: powder for reconstitution 250 mg, 500 mg, 1 g

A prescription stating the dose as 250 mg amoxicillin could mean that the prescriber wants capsules, suspension or injection. In such a situation the pharmacist would need to make a judgement or query the prescriber's intentions.

Doses based on units of formulations

Solid formulations

Examples of units of solid dosage forms are tablets, capsules, sachets and suppositories. The doses of such pharmaceutical products may be expressed as one or more units. Such doses may form part of a dosage regimen, e.g. two tablets at night for 3 days.

Some solid formulations may contain one or more active ingredients, e.g. Rifater tablets contain rifampicin, isoniazid and pyrazinamide, in which case the dose is normally expressed as units of the dosage form, e.g. six tablets daily.

Common examples of a number of active drugs in one dosage unit are the compound analgesics and compound antibiotics:

co-codaprin (aspirin and codeine phosphate)

co-codamol (codeine phosphate and paracetamol)

co-dydramol (paracetamol and dihydrocodeine tartrate)

co-amoxiclav (amoxicillin and clavulanic acid)

co-fluampicil (flucloxacillin and ampicillin).

The calculations involving such unit doses are relatively simple and are normally concerned with calculating a total number of dose units for a specific treatment period.

Example 7.1

Calculate the total number of tablets to be dispensed if a prescription requires two tablets of drug X three times a day for 7 days.

Number of tablets per day is:

$2 \times 3 = 6$

Number of tablets for 7 days is:

$6 \times 7 = 42$

42 tablets should be dispensed.

Some prescribers specify the number of days of treatment by using abbreviations. For example:

- days may be expressed as a fraction of a week, so 3 days will be represented as 3/7 and 5 days as 5/7
- weeks may be represented as a fraction of the number of weeks in the year, so 2 weeks will be written as 2/52 and 6 weeks as 6/52
- months may be represented as a fraction of the number of months in a year, so 6 months will be written as 6/12 and 9 months as 9/12. In the UK, when a month is used like this it generally represents 28 days

If a prescriber uses such an abbreviation, the calculation of the total number of dose units follows the same method as previously.

Example 7.2

A prescription requires two suppositories of drug Y daily for 3/7. How many suppositories should be supplied?

Number of suppositories per day = 2.

3/7 is the abbreviation for 3 days.

Total number of suppositories for 3 days is:

$2 \times 3 = 6$

Six suppositories should be supplied.

Oral liquid formulations

The normal unit of measurement for oral liquid medicines is the 5-mL spoon or multiples thereof. Some medicinal products have a dose or dose range larger than 5 mL. For example, magnesium trisilicate mixture has a dose range of 10–20 mL three times a day. Such a dose range will need to be converted into units of 5 mL, i.e. two to four 5-mL spoonfuls three times a day.

With doses of oral liquid medicines it is important not to confuse 5-mL doses with the total volume of medicine to be supplied.

Example 7.3

A prescription requires a patient to receive a quantity of indigestion mixture with a dosage regimen of 15 mL four times a day for 5 days. How many 5-mL spoonfuls of the mixture will the patient require to take for each dose? Calculate the number of doses and the total volume that should be supplied to the patient.

The patient is prescribed 15 mL as the dose and so will need to take three 5-mL spoonfuls for each dose.

Total number of doses for 5 days is:

$$4 \times 5 = 20$$

Total volume to be supplied is the number of doses multiplied by the dose volume:

$$20 \times 15\,\text{mL} = 300\,\text{mL}$$

The pharmacist needs to dispense 300 mL, which is a total of 20 doses.

In some situations it may be necessary to calculate the length of time taken to use up the total volume of medicine supplied. Such a situation is illustrated in Example 7.4.

Example 7.4

A patient buys a 100-mL bottle of antihistamine mixture to take on holiday. The dosage regimen is two 5-mL spoonfuls four times a day. The patient asks 'If I take the mixture according to the instructions, for how many days will the mixture last?'

The dosage regimen is two 5-mL spoonfuls (that is 10 mL) four times a day, therefore the total volume used per day is 40 mL. The total volume of mixture supplied to the patient is 100 mL, therefore the number of

(continued)

days the mixture will last for is:

$$\frac{100}{40} = 2.5$$

The mixture will be used up by the end of two and a half days.

Dose volumes less than 5 mL

If a patient requires less than 5 mL as a dose, then measuring an accurate dose using a 5-mL spoon would be difficult. Such doses of less than 5 mL may be given using a 5-mL oral syringe. The 5-mL oral syringe is calibrated into 0.5 mL divisions from 1 mL to 5 mL.

Thus, it is possible to deliver volumes between 1 and 5 mL using an oral syringe. The volumes delivered by an oral syringe are usually used for children or very frail adult patients. Example 7.5 demonstrates the calculation of the total volume to be dispensed when a dose volume of less than 5 mL is prescribed.

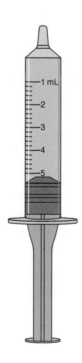

Example 7.5

A very young child is prescribed 2.0 mL of an analgesic suspension three times a day for 4/7. How many millilitres of suspension should the pharmacist dispense?

Volume used per day is:

2.0 mL × 3 = 6.0 mL

4/7 means 4 days, so the total volume used is:

4 × 6 mL = 24 mL

The pharmacist should dispense 24 mL.

Doses based on the weight of drug

Solid formulations

The dose of a drug, in most official publications, is a specified weight or weight range, e.g. codeine phosphate: dose by mouth 30–60 mg. The stated dose may be accompanied by other instructions such as time intervals between doses, specified times of administration, length of treatment, etc. For example, the dose of codeine phosphate is further expanded to: by mouth 30–60 mg every 4 hours, when necessary, to a maximum of 240 mg daily.

Many drugs are available in one or more formulations and may be available in one or more strengths. For example, codeine phosphate is available as a 15-, 30- and 60-mg tablet, as an injection containing 60 mg per millilitre and as a syrup containing 25 mg in 5 mL. A pharmacist may therefore be required to convert a dose of a drug into an equivalent number of tablets, syrup or another dosage form.

Example 7.6

A prescription requires a patient to receive 20 mg domperidone (in tablet form) every 8 hours for 4 weeks. How many tablets should the pharmacist dispense?

(continued)

Domperidone tablets are available only as 10-mg tablets, so, in order for the patient to receive a dose of 20 mg, he or she will need to take two 10-mg tablets. Every 8 hours is equivalent to three times a day, so the patient will need to take six tablets per day.

Four weeks is:

$$4 \times 7 \text{ days} = 28 \text{ days}$$

Total number of 10-mg tablets is:

$$6 \times 28 = 168$$

The pharmacist should dispense 168 tablets.

On occasions, two strengths of the same medicinal product have to be used to obtain the correct dose. Example 7.7 demonstrates such a situation.

Example 7.7

A patient requires 8 mg of drug X per day for 1 week followed by 7 mg of drug X per day for the next week. Drug X is available in tablets of 1 mg and 4 mg. How many tablets of each strength should the pharmacist supply?

8 mg of drug X could be supplied by two 4-mg tablets, so 1 week's supply would consist of fourteen 4-mg tablets.

7 mg of drug X could be supplied by one 4-mg tablet and three 1-mg tablets, so 1 week's supply would consist of seven 4-mg tablets and twenty-one 1-mg tablets.

Thus, the total quantities supplied by the pharmacist should be twenty-one 4-mg tablets and twenty-one 1-mg tablets.

In Examples 7.6 and 7.7 only tablets have been used to illustrate the basic calculations. However, in practice similar calculations could involve suppositories, capsules, powders or other solid dosage forms.

Liquid formulations

Liquid formulations may be prescribed using the weight of the drug as the dose. For example, a prescription may state: 250 mg of paracetamol to be taken twice a day supplied as a suspension. Paracetamol oral suspension contains 250 mg of paracetamol in each 5 mL. Thus, each dose would be 5 mL and the patient would be instructed to take one 5-mL spoonful twice a day.

If the dose is expressed as the weight of drug, then, in the case of a liquid formulation, the dose taken by the patient may be 5 mL or a multiple thereof. Example 7.8 illustrates such a situation.

Example 7.8

A prescription requires 360 mg of paracetamol to be taken four times a day for 3 days, supplied as paediatric paracetamol 120 mg/5 mL suspension. Calculate the volume of paracetamol suspension to be supplied.

First it is necessary to find out what volume of suspension contains 360 mg of paracetamol. We know that the suspension contains 120 mg/5 mL.

Let the unknown volume of suspension that contains 360 mg be y. Setting up proportional sets:

| weight of paracetamol (mg) | 360 | 120 |
| volume of suspension (mL) | y | 5 |

$$\frac{y}{360} = \frac{5}{120}$$

$$y = \frac{5 \times 360}{120}$$

$$y = 15$$

The volume of suspension that contains 360 mg is 15 mL, so a dose of 15 mL four times a day for 3 days would need to be supplied. The total volume to be supplied is:

$$15 \times 4 \times 3 = 180 \, mL$$

If a liquid formulation is prescribed for a very frail person or a very young child, the dose required may be less than 5 mL. Example 7.9 demonstrates such a situation.

Example 7.9

A prescription requires a dose of 200 mg of paracetamol. What volume of paracetamol suspension (250 mg/5 mL) would provide a dose of 200 mg?

We know that paracetamol suspension contains 250 mg/5 mL.
    Let the unknown volume of suspension be *y*. Setting up proportional sets:

weight of paracetamol (mg)   250   200

volume of suspension (mL)   5   *y*

$$\frac{y}{200} = \frac{5}{250}$$

$$y = \frac{5 \times 200}{250}$$

$$y = 4$$

4 mL of paracetamol suspension contains 200 mg of paracetamol.

Injections are another form of liquid formulation. In some situations the dose required may be expressed as a weight and thus the dose will have to be converted to a suitable volume, as in Example 7.10.

Example 7.10

A patient requires an intramuscular injection of 0.5 mg of adrenaline. Adrenaline is available as an injection containing 100 micrograms/mL. How many millilitres of injection will supply the required dose?
(Note: do not confuse micrograms with milligrams.)

First convert 0.5 mg to micrograms using the place value approach:

	mg	–	–	micrograms	
0.5 mg =	0	5	0	0	= 500 micrograms

$\rightarrow$

Let the required volume of adrenaline injection be y. Setting up proportional sets:

weight of adrenaline (micrograms)   100   500

volume of injection (mL)   1 y

$$y = \frac{500}{100}$$

$$y = 5\,mL$$

The patient should receive 5 mL of adrenaline injection, which will contain 0.5 mg (500 micrograms) of adrenaline.

Checking for an overdose

When reviewing a prescription for a patient, it is important to ensure that the patient is receiving the right drug at the right dose. To check that the dose is correct, a pharmacist will need to check the dose against the recommended doses in the BNF and against the maximum dose.

The maximum dose that a patient may take is expressed in different ways in the BNF.

There may be a normal dose or normal dose range stated either in milligrams (for example, mefanamic acid dose in an adult is 500 mg three times a day) or as a number of tablets (for example, co-codaprin 8/400 has a maximum of 8 tablets daily), or as a dose. The stated dose on the prescription should be checked to identify if it fits in that range.

Sometimes a maximum dose to be taken each day or each week is also stated, for example, bisoprolol fumarate has a maximum daily dose of 10 mg. This maximum dose can then be qualified to say that it is given in divided doses or further qualified to state the number of divided doses. If a patient was prescribed *Cardicor* tablets as 7.5 mg tablets, three to be taken each day, then the patient would receive $3 \times 7.5\,mg = 22.5$ mg each day, which would be a potential overdose as it exceeds the maximum dose of 10 mg daily.

Doses in renal impairment

Many drugs are excreted by the kidney either as the drug or its metabolites. A reduction in the function of the kidney may mean that the dose of the drug needs to be reduced.

Chronic kidney disease in adults: the UK guidelines for identification, management and referral (March 2006) define renal function as follows:

Degree of impairment = eGFR mL/minute/1.73 m

Calculation of estimated creatinine clearance in a patient can be done using the Cockcroft and Gault formula, which is stated in the BNF:

Estimated creatinine clearance in mL/minute

$$= \frac{(140 - \text{age}) \times \text{ weight} \times \text{constant}}{\text{serum creatinine}}$$

where
age is in years

weight should be the ideal body weight in kilograms

constant = 1.23 for a man and 1.04 for a woman

serum creatinine is micromol/L.

Doses based on units

The doses of some drugs, usually large biological molecules, are expressed in units rather than weights. Such large molecules are difficult to purify and so, rather than use a weight, it is more accurate to use the biological activity of the drug, which is expressed in units. Examples of such drugs are some hormone products, insulin and a small number of anti-infective drugs.

The calculation of doses and their translation into suitable dosage forms are similar to the calculations elsewhere in this chapter.

Example 7.11

Nystatin has a recommended oral dose for adults of 500 000 units every 6 hours for the treatment of candidiasis. A suspension containing 100 000 units/mL is available. What is the total daily dose of nystatin for an adult and what quantity of suspension would be required for 5 days of treatment?

$\rightarrow$

The adult dose is 500 000 units every 6 hours (in other words four times a day), which is 500 000 × 4 = 2 000 000 units units per day.

The suspension contains 100 000 units/mL. Each dose is 500 000 units, so each dose of suspension would be 5 mL.

Again the patient requires four doses per day, which is 4 × 5 mL = 20 mL, so the total volume of suspension for 5 days = 5 × 20 = 100 mL.

Example 7.12 is another example in which the dose is expressed in units.

Example 7.12

A type of vitamin oral drops contain 5000 units/mL of vitamin A. There are 40 drops/mL. How many drops will provide a child with 750 units of vitamin A?

Let x equal the number of drops. Setting up proportional sets:

units of vitamin A	5000	750
oral vitamin drops	40	x

$$\frac{x}{750} = \frac{40}{5000}$$

$$x = \frac{40 \times 750}{5000}$$

$$x = 6$$

Therefore, 6 drops of oral vitamin drops will contain 750 units of vitamin A.

Vitamins are often expressed in units, or international units (IU) and in grams. This is particularly true for the fat-soluble vitamins: A, D and E. In order to convert from IU to grams or vice versa we need the equivalent values:

Vitamin A	1 IU = 0.344 micrograms (as retinyl acetate)
Vitamin D (ergocalciferol)	40 IU = 1 microgram

Example 7.13

Product A contains 8 mg of vitamin A (as retinyl acetate) and 400 IU of ergo-calciferol and product B contains 2500 IU of vitamin A and 10 micrograms of vitamin D. Which product contains the most vitamins?

First convert the vitamin A in product A from 8 mg to IU.

Remember 1 IU is 0.344 micrograms, so it is necessary to convert the 8 mg to micrograms using the place value approach.

8 mg = 8000 micrograms

Let the vitamin A expressed as IU be y. Setting up proportional sets:

| amount of vitamin A (micrograms) | 0.344 | 8000 |
| number of IU of vitamin A | 1 | y |

$$y = \frac{8000}{0.344}$$

$$= 23\,256\,\text{IU}$$

Therefore, the amount of vitamin A in product A is 23 256 IU.

Next convert the 400 IU of ergocalciferol in product A to micrograms. Let the number of micrograms of ergocalciferol in product A be x. Setting up proportional sets:

| amount of ergocalciferol (micrograms) | 1 | x |
| number of IU of ergocalciferol | 40 | 400 |

$$x = \frac{400}{40}$$

$$x = 10$$

Therefore, there are 10 micrograms of ergocalciferol (vitamin D) in product A.

Comparing the amounts of vitamin A in the two products shows that products A and B contain 23 256 IU and 2500 IU of vitamin A, respectively. Comparison of the amounts of vitamin D in products A and B shows that both products contain the same amount (10 micrograms) of vitamin D. Therefore, product A contains the most vitamins.

Answers are given at the end of the chapter.

Q1   A patient is prescribed two tablets of drug A four times a day for 3 months. How many tablets of drug A should the pharmacist dispense?

Q2   A customer buys an over-the-counter pack of 100 vitamin capsules. The dosage regimen is one capsule three times a day. How many days will the pack last if the customer takes the capsules according to the dosage regimen?

Q3   An inhaler contains 200 metered doses. If the patient inhales two doses three times a day, how long will the inhaler last?

Q4   A patient is prescribed analgesic suppositories to be used six times a day for 5 days, then three times a day for 3 days. How many suppositories should the pharmacist dispense?

Q5   A patient going to a high-risk malaria area requires 8 weeks' treatment. Two different antimalarial tablets are prescribed, A and B. Drug A has a dosage regimen of one tablet per week and drug B has a dosage regimen of two tablets daily. How many tablets of A and B should be supplied to cover the period that the patient is in the malaria area?

Q6   A residential home buys a 1000 pack of senna tablets. Each resident is given two tablets each night. There are 35 residents. How long will it take to use all the senna tablets?

Q7   A prescription for charcoal sachets reads:

Two sachets three times a day for 1/12

How many sachets should be supplied?

Q8   A prescription for drug Y reads:

Three capsules twice a day for 3/7

Two capsules twice a day for 3/7

One capsule twice a day for 2/52

How many capsules should the pharmacist dispense?

Q9 A sachet of physiological 0.9% saline solution is used to bathe an eye. A patient is instructed to bathe both eyes twice a day for 1/12. How many sachets should be supplied to the patient?

Q10 A patient is going on holiday for 3 weeks. He is supplied with 168 tablets of drug C. The dosage regimen is two tablets four times a day. Will the patient have sufficient tablets for the duration of his holiday?

Q11 A patient uses nicotine patches at the rate of one patch every 3 days. How many patches will the patient require for 3 months?

Q12 A patient pack of a drug contains 56 tablets. If the dosage regimen is one tablet four times a day for 4 weeks, how many packs should the pharmacist supply?

Q13 A patient pack of a drug contains 84 tablets and is designed to last for 1 month. If the patient takes one dose twice a day, what is the dose?

Q14 How many 5-mL doses are contained in 120 mL of mixture?

Q15 A patient is required to use 30 mL of mouthwash twice a day. What volume of mouthwash should the pharmacist supply for a 14-day course of treatment?

Q16 A prescription for an indigestion mixture reads:

15 mL four times a day for 2/52

How much mixture should the pharmacist dispense?

Q17 How many 15-mL doses are contained in 240 mL of mixture?

Q18 A patient takes 10 mL of laxative solution at night. What volume will the patient use in a month?

Q19 A mother buys a 150-mL bottle of cough elixir. She gives each of her two children 5 mL four times a day for 3 days. How many doses will be left at the end of 3 days?

Q20 A prescription for a young child reads:

2.5 mL three times a day for 4/7

What volume of drug should the pharmacist dispense?

Q21 A patient requires 7.5 mL of a mixture to be taken four times a day for 3/52. What volume of mixture should be supplied?

Q22 A patient pack contains 30 mL of a syrup. How many days will the syrup last for if the dose is 0.5 mL three times a day?

Q23 A scored tablet containing 100 mg of drug X is available. A prescription for drug X reads:

50 mg three times a day for 10 days

How many tablets should the pharmacist dispense?

Q24 Drug Z is only available as a capsule containing 62.5 mg. A prescription reads:

125 mg four times a day for 1/12

How many capsules of drug Z should the pharmacist dispense?

Q25 Drug A is available as a tablet containing 500 micrograms. A patient requires 2 mg of drug A four times a day for 3/7 and 1.5 mg of drug A for 5/7. How many tablets of drug will be required for a dose of 2 mg and a dose of 1.5 mg? Calculate the total number of tablets to be dispensed to fill the prescription.

Q26 A prescription for drug B reads:

500 mg twice a day for 5 days

Drug B is available as a capsules containing 250 mg. How many capsules should be dispensed to fill the prescription?

Q27 Drug A is available as 2.5-mg and 5-mg tablets. A prescription for drug A requires:

7.5 mg three times a day for 5 days, then

5 mg four times a day for 3 days, then

5 mg twice a day for 3 days, then

2.5 mg three times a day for 7 days.

Calculate how many tablets of 5 mg and 2.5 mg are required to fill the prescription.

Q28 A prescription for drug Z reads:

62.5 mg three times a day for 5 days

Drug Z is available as a suspension containing 250 mg/5 mL. Calculate the volume of each dose and calculate the volume of suspension that should be supplied to the patient.

Q29 A prescription for drug X reads:

240 mg four times a day. Send 100 mL of mixture

Drug X is available as a mixture containing 120 mg/5 mL. Calculate for how many days the mixture will last, assuming that the mixture is taken according to the dosage regimen.

Q30 A solution contains 500 units/mL and the pack size is 25 mL. A patient is given 2500 units three times a day for 5 days. How many packs should the pharmacist dispense for the patient?

Q31 Drug A is available as an elixir containing 150 mg/5 mL. A prescription reads:

225 mg four times a day for 7 days

What volume of the elixir should the pharmacist supply?

Q32 A patient requires 15 mg of morphine sulfate by subcutaneous injection every 4 hours for 16 hours. Morphine sulfate injection is available as 20 mg/mL. What volume of injection should be given on each dosing occasion? What is the total quantity of morphine sulfate given over the 16 hours?

Answers

A1	672	**A7**	168
A2	33.3 rounded to 33 days	**A8**	58
A3	33.3 rounded to 33 days	**A9**	112
A4	39		
		A10	Yes
A5	8 tablets of drug A 112 tablets of drug B	**A11**	28
A6	14.28 rounded to 14 days	**A12**	2

A13   1.5 tablets

A14   24

A15   840 mL

A16   840 mL

A17   16

A18   280 mL

A19   6

A20   30 mL

A21   630 mL

A22   20 days

A23   15

A24   224

A25   4, 3, 63

A26   20

A27   Thirty-three 5-mg tablets
Thirty-six 2.5-mg tablets

A28   1.25-mL dose
18.75 mL total volume

A29   2.5 days

A30   Three

A31   210 mL

A32   0.75 mL per dose
75 mg (every 4 hours for 16 hours is five doses)

8

Doses in children

Learning objectives

By the end of this chapter you will be able to:

- fulfil the learning objectives in Chapter 7
- understand that doses for children can be based on age ranges, weight or body surface area

Doses based on age

The BNF uses ranges:

- First month (neonate)
- Up to 1 year (infant)
- 1 to 6 years would be a dose for a child from 1 year up to their 6th birthday.
- 6 to 12 years

In the *BNF for Children* a number of different ranges are stated depending on the medication.

Doses based on body weight

Many drugs are potent and the dose of such drugs will take into account the body weight of the person receiving the drug. This is particularly important for children. Unless the age is specified, the term 'child' in the BNF includes those who are 12 years and under. Children's doses are expressed in a number of different ways. The doses are usually given for age ranges and can be given as an amount of drug to be given, or the amount of drug to be given can be related to the body weight in kg or body surface area in m^2 of the child or adult. The way that children respond to drugs is different from the adult response. This is particularly true of neonates and both the BNF and the *BNF for Children* advise care in calculating doses for neonates. The advice also states that 'for most drugs the adult maximum dose should not be exceeded'. The example given is if a drug has a dose of 8 mg/kg and a maximum dose of 300 mg a 10-kg child would be given 80 mg but a child weighing 40 kg should receive 300 mg and not 320 mg. It also advises that in overweight children it may be more appropriate to calculate the dose from the ideal weight for a child of that age and height to avoid giving higher doses than required.

Average body weights appear both in the BNF and in the *BNF for Children* as well as information about average heights. The information related to average weights and heights has been reproduced in Table 8.1 and it can be seen that the average man is considered to have a body weight of 68 kg and the average woman to have a body weight of 58 kg, although there will be considerable variation about these average weights. The body weights of children can also be obtained from Table 8.1.

Table 8.1   Age and related body weight and height

Age	Ideal body weight (kg)	Height (cm)
Full-term neonate	3.5	51
1 month	4.3	55
2 months	5.4	58
3 months	6.1	61
4 months	6.7	63
6 months	7.6	67
1 year	9	75
3 years	14	96
5 years	18	109
7 years	23	122
10 years	32	138
12 years	39	149
14-year-old boy	49	163
14-year-old girl	50	159
Adult male	68	176
Adult female	58	164

For example, a 6-month-old child with an average body weight would weigh 7.6 kg and a 5-year-old child with an average body weight would weigh 18 kg. If the child's age is not given in the table, it is usual to estimate the body weight using the weights on either side of the age of the child or to take into account the height of the child. For example, the body weight of a 4-year-old child would be estimated to be between that of a 3 year old and that of a 5 year old, i.e. about 16 kg.

If a baby is born prematurely then calculations of age will have to take into consideration chronological age together with the number of weeks' gestation at birth and are beyond the scope of this book.

The calculation of a dose based on body weight may produce a value that does not correspond to an available dosage form. Example 8.1 illustrates such a situation.

Example 8.1

The recommended dose of fluconazole for mucosal candidiasis in children is 3 mg/kg daily. Calculate the dose of fluconazole for a child aged 3 years and a child aged 11 years. Suggest a suitable formulation for both.

The 3-year-old child
From Table 8.1, a 3-year-old child weighs 14 kg.
  Let the daily dose in milligrams be y. Setting up proportional sets:

dose of fluconazole (mg)	3	y
body weight (kg)	1	14

$y = 3 \times 14$

$y = 42$

The daily dose for a 3-year-old child is 42 mg.

  This dose has to be translated into a suitable formulation for a child. The available formulations of fluconazole are capsules of 50, 150 and 200 mg, and suspensions containing fluconazole 50 mg/ 5 mL and 200 mg/5 mL. Clearly, if the recommended dose is 42 mg, then the capsules are not suitable. (Also remember that a 3-year-old child may not be able to swallow capsules. In fact the *BNF for Children* states that 'Children under 5 years [and some older children] find a liquid

(continued)

formulation more acceptable than tablets or capsules'.) The suspension is a suitable product, but a 5-mL dose contains 50 mg of fluconazole. It is therefore necessary to calculate the volume of suspension that contains the correct dose.

Let the required volume of fluconazole suspension (mL) be y. Setting up proportional sets:

dose of fluconazole (mg)	42	50
volume of suspension (mL)	y	5

$$\frac{y}{42} = \frac{5}{50}$$

$$y = \frac{5 \times 42}{50}$$

$$y = 4.2$$

The child should be given 4.2 mL of fluconazole suspension per day.

The 11-year-old child
Table 8.1 gives weights only for a 10 year old and a 12 year old, so the body weight has to be estimated. In this case the estimate is about 35 kg.

Let the daily dose of fluconazole (mg) be z. Setting up proportional sets:

daily dose of fluconazole (mg)	3	z
body weight (kg)	1	35

$$z = 105$$

The daily dose for an 11-year-old child is 105 mg.

Again it is necessary to translate this dose into a suitable formulation. As the body weight of the child was estimated, it is possible to reduce (or round off) the dose to a convenient 100 mg. In this situation an 11-year-old child might be capable of swallowing a capsule, depending on the medical condition. For a dose of 105 mg it would be possible to provide the child with two 50-mg capsules. Alternatively, a 10-mL dose of the suspension containing 50 mg/5 mL could be given.

Example 8.1 used a drug with a daily dose. Some drugs need to be given at more frequent intervals, as in Example 8.2.

Example 8.2

The dose of co-trimoxazole by intravenous infusion is 36 mg/kg daily in two divided doses for children. Calculate the dose for a 5-year-old child and recommend a suitable dosage form.

From Table 8.1, a 5-year-old child weighs 18 kg.
 Let the daily dose in milligrams be y. Setting up proportional sets:

daily dose of co-trimoxazole (mg)	36	y
body weight (kg)	1	18

$$y = 36 \times 18$$

$$y = 648$$

The daily dose is 648 mg. This daily dose has to be converted into two doses per day, i.e. 648 mg divided by 2, which is 324 mg. The dosage regimen is therefore 324 mg twice a day.
 The available formulation of co-trimoxazole is a sterile solution containing 96 mg/mL. Let the required volume be y. Setting up proportional sets:

volume of sterile solution (mL)	1	y
dose of co-trimoxazole (mg)	96	324

$$y = \frac{324}{96}$$

$$y = 3.375$$

The child should be given 3.375 mL of co-trimoxazole sterile solution as an intravenous infusion twice a day.

Example 8.3 shows another example in which the dose of injectable drugs may be calculated using body weight.

Example 8.3

The drug amikacin has a dose of 15 mg/kg daily in two divided doses for children. Calculate the dose for a 6-month-old child and the volume of paediatric injection to be given.

From Table 8.1, a 6-month-old child weighs 7.6 kg. Let the required dose be y. Setting up proportional sets:

dose of amikacin (mg)	15	y
body weight (kg)	1	7.6

$$y = 7.6 \times 15$$

$$y = 114$$

The dose of amikacin is 114 mg.
   The paediatric injection contains amikacin 50 mg/mL.
   Let the required volume of injection be z. Setting up proportional sets:

volume of injection (mL)	1	z
amount of amikacin (mg)	50	114

$$z = \frac{114}{50}$$

$$z = 2.28$$

2.28 mL of injection should be administered every day in two divided doses, each of 1.14 mL.

Doses based on body surface area

Many physiological phenomena correlate to body surface area and for this reason some doses are calculated using body surface area. In this approach the dose is expressed as the quantity of drug per square metre of body surface area. Examples of such drugs are methotrexate, zidovudine (children only) and lomustine. Paediatric doses may be estimated more accurately using the body surface area method. The calculation of doses using body surface area must of necessity involve determining or obtaining the body surface area. The tables in Appendix 5 show the body surface areas for different weights as taken from the *BNF for Children*. More accurate estimates of body surface area can be obtained using published nomograms.

The method of calculation of doses using body surface area is similar to that using body weight. In other words, the body surface area must be found from the tables before the dose can be calculated, then a suitable dosage form must be found that will deliver the dose. If the weight of the child is not known then you could use Table 8.1 to identify the ideal weight first.

Example 8.4

Calculate the oral dose of methotrexate suitable for a 5-year-old child who weighs 18 kg. The oral dose of methotrexate is 15 mg/m² weekly.

The body surface area of a 5-year-old child weighing 18 kg is 0.74 m². Let the weekly dose of methotrexate be y. Setting up proportional sets:

dose of methotrexate (mg)	15	y
body surface area (m²)	1	0.74

$$y = 15 \times 0.74$$

$$y = 11.1$$

Therefore, the weekly dose of methotrexate is 11.1 mg.

If a paediatric dose is not available for a drug, then prescribers should seek advice from a medicines information centre rather than attempting to calculate a child's dose on the basis of doses used in adults. However, remember that, if a paediatric dose is not available, that drug is probably not licensed for use in children. If the weight of the child is not known it can be looked up in Table 8.1 and then translated to a body surface area in the tables in Appendix 5.

Example 8.5

*Calculate the dose of drug X for a 3-year-old boy if the dose is 120 mg/m²
each day.*

The weight of a 3 year old from Table 8.1 is 14 kg. The surface area
for a weight of 14 kg is 0.62 m². Let the required paediatric dose be y.
Setting up proportional sets:

dose (mg)		y	120
body surface area (m²)		0.62	1

$$\frac{y}{0.62} = \frac{120}{1}$$

$$y = \frac{120 \times 0.62}{1}$$

$$y = 74.4$$

The required dose for the child is 74.4 mg daily.

Practice calculations

Q1   The dose of morphine sulfate for a 6-month-old child by subcutaneous injection is 200 micrograms/kg. Calculate the quantity of
morphine sulfate required for one dose. What volume of injection
should be administered, assuming that it is available in a concentration
of 10 mg/mL?

Q2   Pethidine hydrochloride injection is available in 100 mg/2 mL
ampoules. The recommended dose for a child by intramuscular
injection is 0.5–2 mg/kg. Calculate both extremes of this dose range
for a 12-year-old child. What volume of injection solution should be
administered for both these doses?

Q3   The recommended oral dose for a child of griseofulvin is 10 mg/kg
daily. A suspension containing griseofulvin 125 mg/5 mL is available.
Calculate the dose for a 5-year-old child and the volume of suspension
to be given per dose.

Q4 Using the information in Question 3, calculate the oral dose of griseo-fulvin and the volume of suspension required for a 12-year-old child.

Q5 The recommended dose of didanosine is 120 mg/m² every 12 hours. Calculate the dose and daily dose for a 7-year-old child who weighs 25 kg.

Q6 Drug X has a recommended oral dose for a 6-month-old child of 8 mg/kg twice a day. A suspension is available at a concentration of 40 mg/5 mL. Calculate the dose for a 6-month-old child and recommend the volume of suspension to be administered at each dose.

Q7 The dose of drug X is 75 mg/m². Calculate the dose for a 5-year-old child of average weight.

Q8 Using the data given in Question 7, calculate the dose of drug X for a 10-year-old child of average weight.

Q9 The recommended oral dose of hydroxychloroquine sulfate for a child is 6.5 mg/kg daily. Calculate the dose for a 7-year-old child.

Answers

A1 1.52 mg
0.152 mL

A2 19.5–78 mg
0.39–1.56 mL

A3 180 mg
7.2 mL

A4 390 mg
15.6 mL

A5 110.4 mg
220.8 mg

A6 60.8 mg twice a day
7.6 mL

A7 55.5 mg

A8 82.5 mg

A9 149.5 mg

9

Density, displacement volumes and displacement values

Learning objectives

By the end of this chapter you will be able to:

- express a liquid in either weight or volume using density values
- define and use the term 'displacement value'
- Define and use the term 'displacement volume'
- calculate the amount of base required when making suppositories and pessaries

At 20°C, 1 mL of water weighs 1 g. Thus 1 g of water occupies a volume of 1 mL and so 100 g of water occupies a volume of 100 mL and 1000 mL (1 litre) of water weighs 1000 g (1 kg). This 1 : 1 relationship is considered to hold, for most general pharmaceutical purposes, at the normal ambient temperatures. However, this 1 : 1 relationship between weight and volume is not true for other liquids, solids and semi-solids. For this reason, it is necessary to understand and be able to use the terms 'density', 'displacement volume' and 'displacement values' for some pharmaceutical calculations.

Density

The density of a liquid is the weight per unit volume and is expressed as grams per millilitre. In official references many liquids have their densities expressed as wt/mL, e.g. glycerol has a wt/mL of 1.255–1.26 g. Using the density value it is possible to convert a volume to a weight or a weight to a volume. The conversion to a weight or volume may be for the convenience of the formulator and enables a liquid to be measured as a volume or a weight, whichever is the easiest or most suitable. For example, in the case of a very mobile liquid it may be easier to measure by volume rather than have to weigh the liquid. Alternatively, if the liquid is very viscous, it may be easier to convert a volume to a weight and weigh the viscous liquid.

In the following example a volume is converted to a weight.

Example 9.1

Convert 25 mL of liquid X to its equivalent weight. Liquid X has a weight per mL of 0.65 g.

Let y equal the weight of 25 mL of liquid X. Setting up proportional sets:

| weight (g) | 0.65 | y |
| volume (mL) | 1 | 25 |

$$y = \frac{0.65 \times 25}{1}$$

$$y = 16.25$$

Therefore, 25 mL of liquid X has a weight of 16.25 g.

In the next example a weight is converted into a volume.

Example 9.2

Convert 25 g of liquid Z to its equivalent volume in mL. Liquid Z has a weight per mL of 1.1 g.

$\rightarrow$

Let the volume of liquid Z (mL) be a. Setting up proportional sets:

weight (g)   1.1   25

volume (mL)   1 a

$$a = \frac{1 \times 25}{1.1}$$

$a = 22.73$

Therefore, 25 g of liquid Z has a volume of 22.73 g.

The ability to use density values is needed when a liquid (expressed as a volume) is one of the components of an ointment, cream or gel and the final quantity of the ointment, cream or gel is expressed as a weight. Consider the following example:

Example 9.3

A pharmacist has to prepare 25 g of an ointment to the following formula:

zinc oxide   10 g

liquid paraffin   15 mL

yellow soft paraffin to   100 g

Calculate the final formula for 25 g of the ointment

From the above formula it can be seen that both the solids (zinc oxide and yellow soft paraffin) are expressed as grams and the liquid paraffin is expressed as millilitres (a volume). For all of these ingredients, 1 g does not occupy the volume of 1 mL (or vice versa), and so it is not possible to add volumes of millilitres to quantities in grams to obtain the answer. In order to calculate the final formula, it is necessary to convert the volume of liquid paraffin to a weight using the value for the density of liquid paraffin.

The density of liquid paraffin is 0.88 g/mL.

(continued)

Let the weight of liquid paraffin (g) be z. Setting up proportional sets:

liquid paraffin (g)	z	0.88
liquid paraffin (mL)	15	1

$$z = \frac{0.88 \times 15}{1}$$

$$z = 13.2$$

Therefore, 15 mL of liquid paraffin weighs 13.2 g.

In order to calculate the quantities for 25 g of the ointment, the calculated weight of liquid paraffin will replace the volume of liquid paraffin in the formula.

Note: the quantity of yellow soft paraffin in the formula is to 100 g.

Let the required weight of zinc oxide (g) be x.

Let the required weight of liquid paraffin (g) be y. Setting up proportional sets:

zinc oxide (g)	10	x
liquid paraffin (g)	13.2	y
yellow soft paraffin to (g)	100	25

We can spot that the values in the second column are $\frac{1}{4}$ of those in the first column.

$$x = 2.5$$

$$y = 3.3$$

Therefore, the quantities for 25 g can be written as:

zinc oxide	2.5 g
liquid paraffin	3.3 g
yellow soft paraffin to	25 g

So the weight of yellow soft paraffin required in the formula is:

$$25g - (3.3 + 2.5)g = 19.2g$$

Displacement volumes involving solids in liquids

The definition of displacement volume is the quantity of solvent that will be displaced by a specified quantity of a solid during dissolution (i.e. the preparation of a solution). It is the space or volume of solvent that will be occupied by the solute after a solution has been produced. Knowledge of displacement volumes is required to calculate the volume of a solvent to add to a known amount of solid in order to obtain an exact volume of solution.

The following example may help to explain the concept of displacement volumes.

If we add 5 mL of water to 95 mL of water then we will have a total volume of 100 mL of water. However, if we add 5 g of salt to 95 mL of water and stir the mixture until the salt has dissolved, then we will have a total volume of solution above 95 mL, but it is unlikely to be exactly 100 mL. It may be less than 100 mL or it may be greater. We would need to measure the volume accurately to find out the exact volume. What has happened is that the 5 g of salt dissolves in the water and increases the total volume. In other words the salt will occupy a space and it will displace some of the water, such that the total volume of the solution will be more than 95 mL. This phenomenon by which the salt displaces some of the water and results in an increase in the volume of the resulting solution is important in pharmacy and has resulted in the determination and publication of displacement volumes.

An example of a drug with a known displacement volume is meticillin powder for reconstitution into an injection, which has a displacement volume of 0.7 mL/g. This means that 1 g of meticillin powder will displace (or occupy the space of) 0.7 mL, when it is dissolved in water.

The correct use of displacement volumes is essential when water for injection or another suitable diluent is added to lyophilised drug powder in order to produce an injection solution of a known concentration and volume. For example, the displacement volume of diamorphine is quoted as 0.06 mL/5 mg. This means that 5 mg of diamorphine will displace (or occupy the volume of) 0.06 mL of water. This information can be used to calculate the correct volume of water for injections to add to diamorphine powder to make a known volume of injection solution at a known concentration. This is shown in the following example.

Example 9.4

Calculate the volume of water for injections required to produce 1 mL of an injection containing 5 mg diamorphine. A vial containing 5 mg of diamorphine powder (suitable for reconstitution into an injection) and water for injections is available. The displacement volume of diamorphine is 0.06 mL/5 mg.

The final volume is specified as 1 mL and the volume occupied by the powder is obtained from the displacement volume. The displacement volume is 0.06 mL/5 mg and so the volume occupied by 5 mg of powder will be equivalent to 0.06 mL.

Therefore:

the volume of water required $=$ 1mL $-$ 0.06 mL

$$= 0.94 \text{ mL}$$

Now calculate what would happen if the pharmacist ignored the displacement volume and added 1 mL of water to the powder instead of 0.94 mL.

5 mg of the diamorphine powder displaces 0.06 mL of water. There-fore, if 1 mL of water is added to the powder the total volume of the solution will be:

1 mL $+$ 0.06 mL $=$ 1.06 mL

The difference between 1 mL and 1.06 mL may appear small but it will dilute the concentration of the drug and if the patient were administered 1 mL (as the prescriber requested) then the patient would not receive the correct dose. The dose administered would be 4.7 mg as opposed to the 5 mg requested.

The following example demonstrates the use of a displacement volume in the preparation of an injection.

Example 9.5

A 4-mL injection containing drug X 250 mg/mL is required for a patient. The displacement volume for drug X is 0.56 mL/g. What volume of water for injections should be added to the correct weight of drug X to produce 4 mL of the injection?

The first step is to calculate the amount of drug X in 4 mL of injection. Proportional sets can be used to obtain the answer of 1 g of drug X to be used in the preparation of 4 mL of injection.

The displacement volume of drug X is 0.56 mL/g. Therefore, 1 g of drug X will displace 0.56 mL of solution.

The amount of water for injection required is:

the total volume − displacement volume = 4 − 0.56 = 3.44 mL

Let us try another example, which involves determining the volume required to produce a correct concentration of the drug.

Example 9.6

The displacement volume of drug X is 0.5 mL/50 mg. Drug X is required at a concentration of 2 mg in 1 mL. Calculate the volume of diluent that must be added to 50 mg of drug X to produce the required concentration.

First determine the final volume of the drug solution:
Let the final volume (mL) be y. Setting up proportional sets:

| amount of drug (mg) | 2 | 50 |
| volume (mL) | 1 | y |

$$y = \frac{50}{2}$$
$$y = 25$$

(continued)

Therefore, the final volume of the solution will be 25 mL and this volume will contain 50 mg of drug X.

We know that the volume of diluent required for the reconstitution of drug X is the final volume minus the displacement volume of 50 mg of the drug. Since the displacement volume of drug X is 0.5 mL/50 mg, then

the required volume of diluent $= 25$ mL $- 0.5$ mL

$$= 24.5 \text{ mL}$$

A table of displacement volumes of powder injections is published in *The Pharmaceutical Codex*. This table, however, gives only the displacement volume for one specific quantity of each drug. For example, in the case of diamorphine the displacement volume is that quoted above (0.06 mL/5 mg). Diamorphine is available as a powder for reconstitution in quantities greater than 5 mg. If the prescriber requires more than 5 mg, then these other quantities of powders will need to be used. In such a case it will be necessary to calculate a displacement volume for another quantity of diamorphine.

Example 9.7

Diamorphine is available as a powder for reconstitution in quantities of 30 mg, 100 mg and 500 mg. Using the displacement volume of 0.06 mL/5 mg, calculate how much diluent will be displaced by 30 mg, 100 mg and 500 mg of diamorphine.

Let the volumes (mL) displaced by 30 mg, 100 mg and 500 mg, respectively, be x, y, z. Setting up proportional sets:

volume (mL)	0.06	x	y	z
diamorphine (mg)	5	30	100	500

Spot the relationship between 5 and 30, 100 and 500 to find the values of x, y and z.

→

Alternatively:

$$\frac{0.06}{5} = \frac{x}{30} = \frac{y}{100} = \frac{z}{500}$$

$$x = 0.36$$

$$y = 1.2$$

$$z = 6.0$$

So, 30 mg, 100 mg and 500 mg of diamorphine will displace, respectively, 0.36 mL, 1.2 mL and 6.0 mL of diluent.

Displacement volumes may be used in calculations for different formulations. Many antibiotics are liable to hydrolysis when mixed with water. However, small children cannot take antibiotic tablets/capsules and so, rather than prescribe an antibiotic injection, prescribers may request an antibiotic mixture. Such an antibiotic mixture will have a short time span before the antibiotic is hydrolysed. Thus the pharmacist will prepare the mixture at the time the prescription is presented. Most commercial antibiotic mixture preparations consist of an antibiotic powder mix to which the pharmacist has to add a specific volume of water to produce an exact volume of mixture at a known concentration. This specified volume of water will depend on the manufacturer determining a displacement volume for the antibiotic powder mix (see Example 9.8).

Example 9.8

In order to produce 100 mL of a mixture containing 250 mg of amoxicillin in each 5-mL dose, the pharmacist is required to add 68 mL of water to the antibiotic powder mix. Calculate the displacement volume for a quantity of powder equivalent to 250 mg of amoxicillin.

We need to calculate the total amount of antibiotic in the 100 mL of final mixture.

After reconstitution there will be 250 mg of amoxicillin in 5 mL.

(continued)

Let the total amount of amoxicillin (mg) in 100 mL be y. Setting up proportional sets:

amount of amoxicillin (mg)	250	y
volume (mL)	5	100

$$\frac{y}{100} = \frac{250}{5}$$

$$y = 5000$$

Therefore, 100 mL of the final mixture contains 5000 mg of amoxicillin.

If the pharmacist has to add 68 mL of water to the antibiotic powder mix to produce a final volume of 100 mL, then the antibiotic powder mix must displace 32 mL of water i.e. $(100 - 68\,mL)$.

Thus the antibiotic powder mix contains 5000 mg of amoxicillin and this displaces 32 mL of water.

To calculate the displacement volume of this powder mix, let the volume (mL) displaced by a quantity of antibiotic powder mix equivalent to 250 mg of amoxicillin be x. Setting up proportional sets:

volume (mL)	32	x
antibiotic (mg)	5000	250

$$x = \frac{32 \times 250}{5000}$$

$$x = 1.6$$

Therefore, 1.6 mL of water is displaced by the quantity of antibiotic powder mix containing 250 mg of amoxicillin.

The displacement volume for the antibiotic powder mix is 1.6 mL.

Displacement values involving solids incorporated into other solids

Displacement values are used in calculations when solids are incorporated into another solid. For example, a solid may be mixed intimately with a molten solid, which on cooling forms a solid mix. In a similar way to solids dissolving in a liquid and occupying a volume, so any solid incorporated into another solid will also occupy a volume. Similar weights of different solids may occupy very dissimilar volumes. For example, 1 g of a heavy metal such as mercury will occupy much less volume than 1 g of a fluffy, crystalline powder such as benzoic acid. Thus, solids have densities and this concept of different bulk densities is used in calculations involving the preparation of suppositories and pessaries.

Calculations for suppositories and pessaries

Extemporaneously prepared suppositories and pessaries involve incorporating a drug or drugs into either a waxy or, less frequently, a glycogelatin base. The process involves the use of a mould, so that the size of the suppository is the same irrespective of which base or drug(s) is used in the preparation. The mould will contain a known volume and weight of the base (see below). In the preparation of suppositories the base is mixed with the drug. However, the base and drug may have different bulk densities. So a drug with a low bulk density will displace more of the base than a similar weight of a drug with a high bulk density. In order to ensure that each suppository contains the correct amount of the drug, the bulk densities of the drug have to be taken into account. For many drugs that would be incorporated into a suppository base, the weights of drug that would displace 1 g of the traditional suppository base (theobroma oil) have been calculated and published in *The Pharmaceutical Codex*. These values are referred to as displacement values.

For example, the displacement value of zinc oxide is 4.7. This means that 4.7 g of zinc oxide will displace (or occupy the space of) 1 g of theobroma oil (the suppository or pessary base). In other words, zinc oxide is much more dense than theobroma oil. Another example is menthol which has a displacement value of 0.7. This means that 0.7 g of menthol will displace 1 g of theobroma oil. In this case, menthol is less dense than the suppository base.

In order to calculate the amount of base to be added to the drug to provide the correct amount of drug in each suppository, the displacement value must be used – but note that a displacement value is used only when the drug is expressed as an actual quantity, e.g. x mg or y g. (Suppository and pessary moulds are produced in nominal sizes of 1 g, 2 g, etc. The nominal mould size refers to the quantity of theobroma oil that would occupy the mould. Before use a pharmacist should calibrate the mould by filling with theobroma oil and weighing the suppository produced. The weight of the suppository will indicate the actual size of the mould. If this is substantially different to the nominal value, then the actual value should be used in the calculations shown below.)

Waxy or oily bases

In the section above, theobroma oil was described as the traditional suppository base. Theobroma oil is a natural waxy material, which is solid at room temperature and melts at body temperature, i.e. when inserted into a body cavity. However, in recent years synthetic suppository bases have been developed that have almost replaced the use of theobroma oil. Most of the modern synthetic bases have similar density properties to theobroma oil and so the displacement values determined for drugs incorporated into theobroma oil can be used for the modern synthetic bases.

Displacement values have to be used to calculate the amount of suppository base required when a specified amount of a drug has to be incorporated into a suppository.

Example 9.9

A pharmacist has to prepare six suppositories for a patient, each suppository to be made in a nominal 1-g mould and to contain 0.4 g of bismuth subgallate. Calculate the amount of the base (theobroma oil) that the pharmacist will need to use.

The displacement value of bismuth subgallate is 2.7 and hence 2.7 g of bismuth subgallate will displace 1 g of base. We need to calculate how much bismuth subgallate is required for the six suppositories and how much base will be displaced by that quantity of bismuth subgallate.

Each suppository contains 0.4 g bismuth subgallate.

For six suppositories the total amount of bismuth subgallate will be $6 \times 0.4 = 2.4$ g.

Let the base displaced by 2.4 g of bismuth subgallate be y. Setting up proportional sets:

bismuth subgallate (g)	2.7	2.4
base displaced (g)	1	y

$$y = \frac{1 \times 2.4}{2.7}$$

$$y = 0.89$$

$\rightarrow$

Therefore, 2.4 g of bismuth subgallate will displace 0.89 g of suppository base.

If the pharmacist is preparing six suppositories of 1 g each then the amount of base required will be the amount of base to fill six moulds minus the weight of base displaced by the bismuth subgallate:

$$(6 \times 1 \text{ g}) - 0.89 \text{ g} = 5.11\text{g of base.}$$

Thus the final composition of the suppository mixture will be:

bismuth subgallate	2.4 g
suppository base	5.11 g
total weight	7.51 g

Note: the total weight is greater than the nominal weight of six suppositories, i.e. 6×1 g. This weight difference is because the displacement value of bismuth subgallate is greater than 1.

The following example demonstrates the situation when the displacement value is less than 1.

Example 9.10

Calculate the quantities required to prepare sufficient suppository mixture for twelve 1-g suppositories each containing 50 mg of menthol in theobroma oil. What will each suppository weigh? Assume that the method of preparation means that the pharmacist will need to make an excess of the mixture and so it will be necessary to calculate the quantities for the preparation of 15 suppositories.

The displacement value of menthol is 0.7.

The displacement value is expressed in terms of grams, so the 50 mg dose of menthol has to be converted into grams.

	g	–	–	mg	
50 mg =	0	0	5	0	= 0.05 g

15 suppositories will contain 0.75 g of menthol.

(*continued*)

Let the amount of base displaced by the menthol in 15 suppositories be y. Setting up proportional sets:

mass of menthol (g)	0.7	0.75
base displaced (g)	1	y

$$y = \frac{0.75}{0.7}$$
$$y = 1.1$$

Therefore, 0.75 g of menthol displaces 1.1 g of theobroma base.

So the quantity of theobroma oil required to produce 15 supposi-tories, containing a total of 0.75 g of menthol is:

$$(15 \times 1 \text{ g}) - 1.1 \text{ g} = 13.9 \text{ g}$$

i.e. 13.9 g of theobroma oil is required.

The final formula for 15 suppositories is:

menthol	0.75 g
theobroma oil	13.9 g
total weight	14.65 g

Therefore, each suppository weighs 0.98 g. This is less than the nominal 1 g because of the displacement value for the menthol.

If more than one medicament is included in a suppository, the displacement of the base by both medicaments should be calculated.

Example 9.11

Assume that the menthol suppositories in the above calculation are each to contain 300 mg of paracetamol in addition to the menthol. Calculate the weight of base required to produce the same quantity of suppository mixture.

$\rightarrow$

First calculate the amount of base displaced by the paracetamol.

Each suppository will contain 300 mg (0.3 g) of paracetamol and 15 suppositories will contain $15 \times 0.3\,g = 4.5\,g$ of paracetamol.

Let the amount of base (g) displaced by 4.5 g of paracetamol be b.

The displacement value of paracetamol is 1.5. Setting up proportional sets:

paracetamol (g)	1.5	4.5
base displaced (g)	1	b

$$\frac{b}{4.5} = \frac{1}{1.5}$$
$$b = 3$$

Therefore, 4.5 g of paracetamol displaces 3 g of suppository base.

The amount of base required to produce the suppositories is $(15 \times 1)\,g$ minus the amounts displaced by both the menthol and the paracetamol. Remember that the menthol will displace 1.1 g of base and the paracetamol will displace 3 g.

$$\text{Therefore, weight of base required} = 15\,g - (1.1 + 3)\,g$$
$$= 10.9\,g$$

The total weight of the suppository mixture is:

Menthol	0.75 g
paracetamol	4.5 g
theobroma base	10.9 g
total weight	16.15 g

Therefore, each individual suppository will weigh 1.08 g.

Aqueous suppository bases

If an aqueous base for the preparation of suppositories or pessaries is required, then a glycogelatin base or similar can be used. A drug can be incorporated into the aqueous base and, if a specified quantity per suppository is prescribed, the displacement value of the drug has to be used in calculating the amount of base required.

The glycogelatin base is denser than theobroma oil and the other waxy-type bases: 1.2 g of glycogelatin base occupies the same volume as 1 g of theobroma oil. Thus, when calculating the amount of glycogelatin base required, it is important to take this factor into account. Hence a nominal 1-g mould will hold 1.2 g of glycogelatin base and a 2-g mould will hold 2.4 g.

Example 9.12

A pharmacist has to prepare twenty 2-g glycogelatin pessaries each containing 150 mg miconazole nitrate. The displacement value of miconazole nitrate is 1.6. Assume for ease of preparation that the pharmacist makes sufficient for 25 pessaries.

First calculate the displacement due to the drug.

25 pessaries will contain (25×150) mg of miconazole nitrate $=$ 3750 mg.

Converting milligrams to grams:

	g	–	–	mg	
3750 mg =	3	7	5	0	= 3.75 g

The displacement value for miconazole nitrate is 1.6.

Let the displacement due to the drug be y. Setting up proportional sets:

miconazole (g)	1.6	3.75
base displaced (g)	1	y

$$\frac{y}{3.75} = \frac{1}{1.6}$$

$$y = 2.344$$

Therefore, 3.75 g of miconazole nitrate is required for 25 pessaries and this quantity of drug will displace 2.344 g of base. But the displacement

$\rightarrow$

value is determined for a theobroma oil-type base, not a glycogelatin base.

If 25 theobroma oil pessaries were to be produced then the amount of base required would be:

(25 pessaries × 2 g) − 2.344 g (quantity displaced by the drug)

As 1.2 g of the glycogelatin base is equal to 1 g of the theobroma oil base, the amount of glycogelatin base required is:

1.2 [(25 × 2) − 2.344] g = 57.19 g of glycogelatin base

The final formula for the pessaries will be:

miconazole nitrate	3.75 g
glycogelatin base	57.19 g
total weight	60.94 g

Therefore, each nominal 2-g pessary will weigh 2.44 g.

The difference between the nominal weight of the pessary and the actual weight is mainly due to the weight of the glycogelatin base, because each pessary contains only 150 mg of the drug.

Note: if the quantity of drug to be incorporated into a suppository or pessary is expressed as a percentage it is not necessary to use a displacement value.

Example 9.13

A pharmacist has to prepare 20 g of suppository mixture to the formula:

bismuth oxide	*6%*
hydrocortisone acetate	*1%*
suppository base to	*100%*

In this situation the quantities will be calculated in the usual way.

(continued)

Let the required quantities of bismuth oxide and hydrocortisone acetate (g), be respectively x and y. Setting up proportional sets:

	amount	percentage
bismuth oxide (g)	x	6
hydrocortisone acetate (g)	y	1
suppository base (g) to	20	100

$x = 1.2$

$y = 0.2$

Therefore, the formula for 20 g of suppository mixture will be:

bismuth oxide	1.2 g
hydrocortisone acetate	0.2 g
suppository base to 20 g	18.6 g (i.e. 20 g − 1.2 g − 0.2 g)

Displacement values

Practice calculations

Answers are given at the end of the chapter.

Calculations involving density

Q1   Methyl salicylate has a density of 1.18 g/mL. Calculate the weight of 45 mL of methyl salicylate and calculate the volume occupied by 60 g of methyl salicylate.

Q2   25 g of arachis oil are required to be incorporated into 250 g of ointment base. If the weight per millilitre of arachis oil is 0.917 g, how many millilitres of arachis oil would be equivalent to 25 g?

Q3   Liquid paraffin has a density of 0.91 g/mL. What is the weight of 2 litres? Express your answer in grams and kilograms.

Q4   A pharmacist is required to provide 75 mL of glycerol. A suitable measure is not available. What weight of glycerin is equivalent to 75 mL? Assume that the density of glycerol is 1.25 g/mL.

Q5   If the weight of 40 mL of a liquid is 37.5 g, what is the density of the liquid in g/mL?

Q6   A prescription states:

glycerol	10 mL
drug Z	25 g
ointment base to	100 g

If the density of glycerol is 1.25 g/mL, give the quantities (in grams) of all the ingredients if 60 g of the ointment is required.

Displacement volumes involving solids in liquids

Q7   Drug Z has a negligible displacement volume in water. If 10 mL of water is added to 50 mg of drug Z, what will be the final volume of the solution?

Q8   A pharmacist adds 75 mL of water to 35 g of a soluble drug powder and the volume of the final solution is 115 mL. Calculate the displacement volume of the drug powder.

Q9   Ampicillin powder for reconstitution into an injection has a displacement volume of 0.8 mL/g. If 10 mL of water is added to 500 mg of the powder, calculate the total volume of the solution. What would be the concentration expressed as mg/mL?

Q10   A prescriber requires an injection solution containing vancomycin 50 mg in 1 mL; 500 mg of vancomycin powder for reconstitution into an injection is available in a vial. The displacement volume for the powder is 0.3 mL per 500 mg. What volume of sterile diluent should be added to the vancomycin powder to produce the required concentration? What is the total volume of the final injection solution?

Q11   Drug X has a displacement volume of 0.1 mL/30 units and is required as an injection containing 6 units in 1 mL. Drug X is available as a powder suitable for reconstitution into an injection in a vial containing 90 units. What volume of diluent should be added to the powder to produce the injection solution?

Q12   A drug is required in the concentration 20 mg/mL. Drug powder suitable for preparing the solution is available with a displacement volume of 0.15 mL/100 mg. How much diluent and how much powder should be used to produce 5 mL of a solution of the required concentration?

Calculations for suppositories and pessaries

The following displacement values may be required for the next set of calculations

aspirin	1.1
camphor	0.7
castor oil	1.0
hydrocortisone	1.5
bismuth subgallate	2.7
sulfur	1.6
zinc sulfate	2.4

Q13 Calculate the quantities required to produce 100 suppositories to the following formula:

castor oil	10 mg
zinc sulfate	200 mg

theobroma oil sufficient to produce a 1-g suppository

Q14 Calculate the quantities required to produce 20 pessaries to the following formula:

hydrocortisone	150 mg

waxy pessary base sufficient to produce a 2-g pessary

(assume the pessary base has the same physical characteristics as theobroma oil)

Q15 Twelve nominal 1-g suppositories each containing 100 mg of camphor and 75 mg of aspirin are prescribed for a patient. Calculate the quantities required if the suppository base is theobroma oil. Assume that no excess mixture is prepared.

Q16 Repeat the question above assuming that the suppository base is glycogelatin. What is the weight of each suppository?

Q17 2-g suppositories each containing 125 mg of bismuth subgallate and 50 mg of sulfur in theobroma oil are required to fill a private prescription. Calculate the quantities required of each component to produce 25 suppositories. What is the weight of each suppository?

Q18 A pharmacist has to make a batch of one hundred 1-g suppositories, each containing 75 mg of drug J. Drug J has a displacement value of 2.1. Assuming that the pharmacist makes a 20% excess to allow for losses in preparation and that the base is glycogelatin, calculate the quantities of base and drug J required. What is the final weight of each suppository?

Q19 A prescription reads:

cocaine hydrochloride	10%
theobroma oil to	100%

Send six 1-g suppositories

Assume that the pharmacist needs to make two additional suppositories to those prescribed because of the method of preparation. Calculate the quantities required to make the suppository mix.

Answers

Calculations involving density

A1 45 mL methyl salicylate = 53.1 g
60 g methyl salicylate = 50.85 mL

A2 25 g arachis oil = 27.26 mL

A3 2 litres of liquid paraffin = 1820 g = 1.82 kg

A4 75 mL glycerol = 93.75 g

A5 0.938 g/mL

A6
glycerol	7.5 g
drug Z	15 g
ointment base	37.5 g

Displacement volumes involving solids in liquids

A7   10 mL

A10   volume of diluent = 9.7 mL
total volume = 10 mL

A8   1.14 mL/g

A11   14.7 mL

A9   total volume = 10.4 mL
concentration = 48.1 mg/mL

A12   diluent = 4.85 mL
drug powder = 100 mg

Calculations for suppositories and pessaries

A13
castor oil	1 g
zinc sulfate	20 g
theobroma oil	$100 - (1 + 8.33) = 90.67$ g

A14
hydrocortisone	3 g
base	$40 - \dfrac{3}{1.5} = 38$ g

A15
camphor	1.2 g
aspirin	0.9 g
base	$12 - \dfrac{1.2}{0.7} + \dfrac{0.9}{1.1} = 12 - (1.71 + 0.82) = 9.47$ g

A16   weight of glycogelatin base = $9.47 \times 1.2 = 11.36$
weight of base plus ingredients = $11.36 + 1.2 + 0.9 = 13.46$ g
therefore weight of each suppository = 1.12 g

A17

	for 1 suppos	for 25 suppos
bismuth subgallate	125 mg	3.125 g
sulfur	50 mg	1.25 mg
base	to 2 g	$50 - \dfrac{3.125}{2.7} + \dfrac{1.25}{1.6}$
		$= 50 - (1.157 + 0.781)$
		$= 48.06$ g

$$\text{weight of each suppository} = \frac{48.06 + 3.125 + 1.25}{25} = \frac{52.43}{25} = 2.097 \text{ g}$$

A18

	for 1 suppos	for 120 suppos
drug J	75 mg	9 g
base to	1 g	$120 - \dfrac{9}{2.1} = 115.71$ g

If the base is glycogelatin the required amount will be $1.2 \times 115.71 = 138.85$ g.

$$\text{Weight of each suppository} = \frac{(138.85 + 9)}{120} = 1.232 \text{ g}$$

A19 Mixture sufficient for 8 suppositories will be made, i.e. 8 g
Therefore, cocaine hydrochloride $= 0.8$ g
theobroma oil $= 7.2$ g

10

Calculations involving molecular weights

Learning objectives

By the end of this chapter you will be able to:

- calculate the molecular weight of a drug
- calculate the amount of drug (expressed as the base) in a salt or hydrate of a drug
- use molecular weights to determine the legal classification of drugs
- define the terms 'mole' and 'molar solution'

Many pharmaceutical calculations involve the need to know the molecular weight or molecular structure of the drug. In some cases these can be found in reference books, but on some occasions it may be necessary to work out the molecular weight from the individual atomic weights.

Calculations involving molecular weights are rarely seen in community pharmacy. They are, however, more usual in hospital pharmacy. A common situation when these calculations are used is when a patient has presented with an electrolyte imbalance. Since the electrolyte imbalance will be specific to each patient, a standard intravenous infusion may need to have amounts of various ions, such as potassium, added. Often the amount to be added will be calculated using the molecular weight of the available product.

Molecular weights of drugs

The molecular weight of a drug is the sum of all the atomic weights of the individual atoms in the molecule expressed in grams. For example, a molecule of potassium bromide (KBr) consists of one atom of potassium and one atom of bromine (atomic weights are given in Appendix 4), so the molecular weight of potassium bromide is:

K + Br

$39 + 79.9 = 118.9$ g

If there is more than one atom of the same kind in a molecule, all the individual atoms must be included in the calculation. For example, aluminium chloride ($AlCl_3$) consists of one atom of aluminium and three atoms of chlorine, so the molecular weight of aluminium chloride is:

Al + Cl_3

$27 + (35.5 \times 3) = 133.5$ g

If a molecule has associated water molecules, these must be included in the calculation of molecular weight. For example, the molecular weight of zinc sulfate monohydrate ($ZnSO_4.H_2O$) is:

Zn + S + O_4 + H_2 + O

$65.4 + 32 + (16 \times 4) + (1 \times 2) + 16 = 179.4$ g

The formulae of the above molecules are simple. Many drug molecules have much more complicated formulae and to calculate the molecular weight it is easier to use the empirical formula than the structural formula. For example, the empirical formula of aspirin is $C_9H_8O_4$, so the molecular weight can be calculated as follows:

$(9 \times 12) + (8 \times 1) + (4 \times 16) = 180$ g

The structural formula of aspirin is:

From the structural formula it is not readily clear how many atoms of each element are present. In order to calculate the molecular weight from the structural formula, it is therefore necessary to determine the number of each atom in the empirical formula. However, during the process of converting the structural formula into the empirical formula, it is easy to introduce errors; therefore, wherever possible, if the empirical formula is available it should be used. Empirical and structural formulae of drugs can be found in official publications, e.g. *The Pharmaceutical Codex, Martindale* and pharmacopoeias.

Knowledge of the molecular weight of a compound or drug allows the calculation of the amount of element/base/salt present in that compound or drug. With some drugs, it is only one part of the molecule that is pharmacologically active.

Example 10.1

How many milligrams of sodium ions are contained in a 600-mg tablet of sodium chloride?

First the atomic weights need to be found for each of the elements and then the molecular weight can be calculated:

Na + Cl

$23 + 35.5 = 58.5$

Therefore, the molecular weight of sodium chloride is 58.5 g and the sodium ion represents 23 parts of 58.5 parts of the sodium chloride molecule.

Let the number of milligrams of sodium ions in 600 mg of sodium chloride be x. Setting up proportional sets:

	sodium chloride	sodium
weight (mg)	600	x
molecular/atomic weight	58.5	23

$$\frac{600}{58.5} = \frac{x}{23}$$

$x = 235.9$

Therefore, 235.9 mg of sodium ions are contained in a 600-mg tablet of sodium chloride.

Some pharmaceutical calculations require the percentage of a specific component of a drug to be determined. In such cases it may be necessary to use a knowledge of molecular weights.

Example 10.2

What is the percentage of lithium contained in a 400-mg tablet of lithium carbonate?

First the molecular weight of lithium carbonate must be calculated from the empirical formula and the relevant atomic weights.

$Li_2 + C + O_3$

$(7 \times 2) + 12 + (16 \times 3) = 74$

The molecular weight of lithium carbonate is 74 g. The lithium represents 14 parts of the 74 parts of the lithium carbonate molecule.

Let the number of milligrams of lithium in 400 mg of lithium carbonate be y. Setting up proportional sets:

	lithium	lithium carbonate
amount (mg)	y	400
molecular/atomic weight	14	74

$$\frac{y}{14} = \frac{400}{74}$$

$$y = 75.7$$

400 mg of lithium carbonate contains 75.7 mg lithium. This can be expressed as a percentage:

$$= 18.92\%$$

Alternatively, the percentage of lithium in lithium carbonate can be calculated directly from the ratio of lithium to lithium carbonate using the atomic weights, i.e. bypassing the step involving the calculation of the amount of lithium in lithium carbonate.

$\rightarrow$

Let the required percentage be x. Setting up proportional sets:

	lithium	lithium carbonate
percentage	x	100
molecular/atomic weight	14	74

$$\frac{x}{14} = \frac{100}{74}$$

$$x = 18.92$$

There is 18.92% of lithium in 400 mg of lithium carbonate.

Drugs and their salts

Some drugs may be prepared with different salts attached to the basic drug molecule. For example, iron is presented as a number of different ferrous salts. The ferrous salts that are available for use as drugs are fumarate, gluconate, succinate, sulfate and dried sulfate. Although different salts of a drug may be prescribed, it is normal to give an equivalent amount of the base drug. It such a case it may be necessary to calculate the equivalent amount of base drug in two different salts.

Equivalent amounts of drug in different salts of that drug

In Example 10.3 two salts of iron are compared in terms of their iron content.

Example 10.3

What weight of ferrous gluconate contains the same quantity of iron as a tablet containing 200 mg of ferrous sulfate (dried)?

First let us calculate the molecular weight of ferrous sulfate:

$$Fe + S + O_4$$

$$56 + 32 + (16 \times 4) = 152$$

The molecular weight of ferrous sulfate is 152.

From the above, it can be seen that the iron represents 56 parts of the total 152.

(continued)

Let the amount of iron in 200 mg of ferrous sulfate be y.
Setting up proportional sets:

	Iron	ferrous sulfate
amount (mg)	y	200
molecular/atomic weight	56	152

$$\frac{y}{56} = \frac{200}{152}$$
$$y = 73.68$$

73.68 mg of iron is contained in 200 mg of ferrous sulfate.

Now let us tackle the second part of the problem, namely how much ferrous gluconate contains the same amount of elemental iron as 200 mg of ferrous sulfate. Ferrous gluconate has an empirical formula of $C_{12}H_{22}FeO_{12}.2H_2O$ and a molecular weight of 482. If we look at the empirical formula we can see that it contains one atom of iron, therefore 56 parts of the molecular weight of ferrous gluconate are accounted for by the iron (the atomic weight of iron equals 56). The problem is to calculate how much ferrous gluconate will contain 73.68 mg of iron.

Let the amount of ferrous gluconate be z. Setting up proportional sets:

	ferrous gluconate	iron
amount of iron (mg)	z	73.68
molecular atomic weight	482	56

$$\frac{z}{482} = \frac{73.68}{56}$$
$$z = 634.17$$

634.17 mg of ferrous gluconate contains the same amount of iron as 200 mg of ferrous sulfate.

Calculating the weight of the salt, if the drug is expressed as the base

Many drug preparations consist of the salt (or salts) of a base drug. However, in describing the drug preparation it is usual to express the dose or strength in terms of the base drug rather than the actual salt used in the preparation. One such example is the drug erythromycin. Some of the available formulations of erythromycin are as follows:

- Erythrocin tablets contain 250 mg and 500 mg erythromycin (as stearate).
- The paediatric suspension contains 125 mg, 250 mg and 500 mg of erythromycin (as the ethyl succinate) per 5 mL.
- The intravenous infusion powder is presented as a vial containing 1 g erythromycin (as lactobionate).

In other words, the paediatric suspensions contain an amount of erythromycin ethyl succinate that is equivalent to 125 mg, 250 mg and 500 mg of erythromycin in every 5 mL. The 250-mg and 500-mg erythrocin tablets contain, respectively, the equivalent of 250 mg and 500 mg of erythromycin presented as the stearate.

If the empirical formulae of erythromycin, erythromycin ethyl succinate and erythromycin stearate are known, it is possible to calculate the amount of the erythromycin salt required in each preparation, i.e. to give a known quantity of erythromycin.

The molecular weights are:

erythromycin	734
erythromycin ethyl succinate	862
erythromycin stearate	1018

Example 10.4

Using the above data calculate the amounts of erythromycin ethyl succinate and erythromycin stearate that are equivalent to 250 mg erythromycin.

Let the amount of erythromycin ethyl succinate be x and the amount of erythromycin stearate be y. Setting up proportional sets:

	amount	molecular weight
erythromycin (mg)	250	734
erythromycin ethyl succinate (mg)	x	862
erythromycin stearate (mg)	y	1018

(*continued*)

$$\frac{x}{250} = \frac{862}{734}$$

and

$$\frac{y}{250} = \frac{1018}{734}$$

$x = 294$ and $y = 347$

Therefore, 294 mg of erythromycin ethyl succinate and 347 mg of erythromycin stearate contain the equivalent of 250 mg erythromycin.

Using the same approach the amount of adrenaline acid tartrate in adrenaline injection can be determined.

Example 10.5

Calculate the amount of adrenaline acid tartrate required in each millilitre of adrenaline injection. Adrenaline injection contains 100 micrograms of adrenaline (as the acid tartrate) per mL. The molecular weights of adrenaline and adrenaline acid tartrate are 183 and 333, respectively.

Let the amount of adrenaline acid tartrate be z. Setting up proportional sets:

	amount (micrograms)	molecular weight
adrenaline acid tartrate	z	333
adrenaline	100	183

$$\frac{z}{100} = \frac{333}{183}$$

$z = 182$

Therefore, each millilitre of injection contains 182 micrograms of adrenaline acid tartrate, which is equivalent to 100 micrograms of adrenaline.

Calculations in which the base to salt ratio is more than 1

When some drug bases are converted into a salt the resultant molecule may consist of two or more base units attached to one salt unit. For example, salbutamol has the empirical formula $C_{13}H_{21}NO_3$ and salbutamol sulfate has the formula $(C_{13}H_{21}NO_3)_2.H_2SO_4$. It can be seen that one molecule of salbutamol sulfate contains two molecules of the base and this must be taken into account in calculations as shown in the next example.

Example 10.6

How many grams of salbutamol sulfate will contain the same amount of salbutamol base as 5 g of salbutamol? The molecular weights of salbutamol and salbutamol sulfate are 239 and 577, respectively.

From the empirical formulae we know that salbutamol sulfate contains twice the amount of salbutamol as the base and that salbutamol sulfate is a hydrate. Therefore, two molecules of salbutamol (equivalent mol wt $=(239 \times 2)=478$) contain the same amount of salbutamol base as one molecule of salbutamol sulfate.

Let the amount of salbutamol sulfate containing the same amount of salbutamol base as 5 g of salbutamol be x. Setting up proportional sets:

	amount (g)	equivalent molecular weight
salbutamol sulfate	x	577
salbutamol	5	478

$$\frac{x}{5} = \frac{577}{478}$$

$$x = 6.04$$

Therefore, 6.04 g of salbutamol sulfate contains the same amount of salbutamol base as 5 g of salbutamol.

Using weights of salts expressed as equivalent to a known weight of base

In some official publications the salts of a drug are expressed as an amount equivalent to a known amount of the anhydrous base. For example, the *British National Formulary* (BNF) notes that 'quinine (anhydrous base) 100 mg is equivalent to quinine bisulfate 169 mg is equivalent to quinine dihydrochloride 122 mg is equivalent to 121 mg of quinine sulfate'.

Example 10.7

Using the BNF equivalents for quinine (anhydrous base), quinine bisulfate and quinine dihydrochloride and given that quinine anhydrous base has a molecular weight of 324, estimate the molecular weights of the other two salts using the proportional sets approach.

Let the molecular weights of quinine bisulfate and quinine dihydrochloride be x and y, respectively. Setting up proportional sets:

	equivalents	*molecular weight*
quinine anhydrous base	100	324
quinine bisulfate	169	x
quinine dihydrochloride	122	y

$$\frac{x}{324} = \frac{169}{100}$$

and

$$\frac{y}{324} = \frac{122}{100}$$

$$x = 548 \quad \text{and} \quad y = 395$$

Therefore, the estimated molecular weights for quinine bisulfate and quinine dihydrochloride are 548 and 395, respectively. These weights can be checked using official references.

The equivalent values for the quinine salts can be used to determine the approximate amount of quinine anhydrous base in a tablet containing a quinine salt.

Example 10.8

The BNF states that a 300-mg tablet of quinine bisulfate contains less quinine than a 300-mg tablet of quinine sulfate. By calculation show that this statement is correct. (The BNF equivalent for quinine sulfate is 121.)

$\rightarrow$

Use the equivalent values found in Example 10.7. Let the amount of quinine anhydrous base be x. Setting up proportional sets:

	equivalents	amount (mg)
quinine anhydrous base	100	x
quinine sulfate	121	300

$$\frac{100}{121} = \frac{x}{300}$$

$x = 248$

A quinine sulfate 300-mg tablet contains 248 mg of quinine anhydrous base. Set up proportional sets for quinine bisulfate:

	equivalents	amount (mg)
quinine anhydrous base	100	x
quinine bisulfate	169	300

$$\frac{100}{169} = \frac{x}{300}$$

$x = 178$

A quinine bisulfate 300-mg tablet contains 178 mg of quinine anhydrous base.

Therefore, a quinine bisulfate 300-mg tablets contains less anhydrous quinine than a 300-mg tablet of quinine sulfate and so the BNF statement is correct.

Drugs and their hydrates

Many drugs exist as both the anhydrous form and hydrates. An example is ferrous sulfate, which exists in the anhydrous form and as a hydrate. Thus, equal weights of the anhydrous and the hydrate of ferrous sulfate will contain different amounts of iron. In order to calculate the equivalent amounts of iron, it is necessary to take into account the water of hydration in the molecule.

Example 10.9

1 L of Paediatric Ferrous Sulfate Oral Solution BP contains 12 g of ferrous sulfate. A pharmacist is required to make 150 mL of this solution, but only ferrous sulfate anhydrous is available. How much ferrous sulfate anhydrous should be used?

First we need to calculate how much ferrous sulfate is required to make 150 mL of the preparation.

Let the required amount of ferrous sulfate be *x*. (Remember that 1 L equals 1000 mL.) Setting up proportional sets:

amount of ferrous sulfate (g)	*x*	12
volume of solution (mL)	150	1000

$$\frac{x}{150} = \frac{12}{1000}$$
$$x = 1.8$$

1.8 g of ferrous sulfate is required to make 150 mL of paediatric solution.

The molecular weights of ferrous sulfate and ferrous sulfate anhydrous are 278 and 152, respectively.

Let the required amount of ferrous sulfate anhydrous be *y*. Setting up proportional sets:

	amount (g)	*molecular weight*
ferrous sulfate	1.8	278
ferrous sulfate anhydrous	*Y*	152

$$\frac{y}{1.8} = \frac{152}{278}$$
$$y = 0.984$$

0.984 g of ferrous sulfate anhydrous is equivalent to 1.8 g of ferrous sulfate, so the pharmacist should use 0.984 g of the anhydrous ferrous sulfate in preparing 150 mL of solution.

Another example in which a drug is available in different hydrated forms is codeine phosphate. The *British Pharmacopoeia* directs that 30-mg codeine phosphate tablets contain codeine phosphate or the equivalent amount of codeine phosphate sesquihydrate.

Example 10.10

How much codeine phosphate sesquihydrate is equivalent to 30 mg of codeine phosphate?

If we look at the formulae for both phosphates, it can be seen that Codeine Phosphate BP exists as the hemihydrate and has a molecular weight of 406 and that codeine sesquihydrate has a molecular weight of 424. The difference in the molecular weights is due to one molecule of water, i.e. the difference between a sesqui- and a hemihydrate. We can calculate the amount of codeine phosphate sesquihydrate that is equivalent to 30 mg of codeine phosphate.

Let the amount of codeine phosphate sesquihydrate be z. Setting up proportional sets:

	amount (mg)	molecular weight
codeine phosphate hemihydrate	30	406
codeine phosphate sesquihydrate	z	424

$$\frac{z}{30} = \frac{424}{406}$$

$$z = 31.33$$

A 30-mg codeine phosphate tablet would contain 30 mg of codeine phosphate hemihydrate or 31.33 mg codeine phosphate sesquihydrate.

Calculation of legal classifications using molecular weights

If a drug is available as different salts, then the legal classification of each salt may be based on the equivalent amount of base drug. In the UK, examples of such drugs are pholcodine and its salts, morphine and its salts, hyoscyamine hydrobromide and sulfate, ephedrine hydrochloride and quinine and its salts.

Classification based on maximum dose (calculated as base)

An example of a classification based on maximum dose is ephedrine hydrochloride. Ephedrine hydrochloride is a prescription-only medicine, but if it is in a preparation intended for internal use (other than nasal sprays and drops) with a maximum dose equivalent of 30 mg of ephedrine and a maximum daily dose equivalent of 60 mg of ephedrine, the preparation can be sold over the counter. Therefore, in order to ascertain the legal classification of an ephedrine hydrochloride preparation it is necessary to calculate the equivalent amount of ephedrine base.

Example 10.11

What is the maximum dose and daily dose of ephedrine hydrochloride that can be sold over the counter?

The molecular weight of ephedrine hydrochloride is 202 and the molecular weight of ephedrine is 165.

Let the maximum dose of ephedrine hydrochloride be x and the maximum daily dose of ephedrine hydrochloride be y. Setting up proportional sets:

	ephedrine	ephedrine hydrochloride
molecular/atomic weights	165	202
maximum dose (mg)	30	x
maximum daily dose (mg)	60	y

$$\frac{x}{202} = \frac{30}{165}$$

and

$$\frac{y}{202} = \frac{60}{165}$$

$$x = 36.7 \quad \text{and} \quad y = 73.4$$

A preparation of ephedrine hydrochloride can be sold over the counter provided that the maximum dose and the maximum daily dose do not exceed 36.7 mg and 73.4 mg respectively. If either one or both of these doses are exceeded then the preparation becomes a prescription-only medicine.

Classification based on maximum strength of base

In some legal classifications, the maximum dose is not stipulated but a maximum strength is stated. For example, morphine and its salts are CD POM (Schedule 2), but in the case of the salts, if the morphine cannot be readily recovered in amounts that constitute a risk to health with a maximum strength of 0.2% (calculated as the anhydrous morphine base) the preparation becomes a CD Inv POM (Schedule 5).

In order to determine the legal classification of liquid preparations of morphine salts, it is therefore necessary to calculate the weight of the anhydrous morphine base.

Example 10.12

What is the maximum amount of morphine hydrochloride that can be incorporated into 200 mL of a liquid preparation so that the legal classification is a CD Inv POM?

The molecular weights of anhydrous morphine base and morphine hydrochloride are 285 and 376, respectively. A 0.2% solution will contain 0.2 g in 100 mL and therefore 0.4 g in 200 mL. The equivalent of 0.4 g of anhydrous base (in the form of morphine hydrochloride) is the maximum amount allowed in the liquid preparation, if it is to be classified as a CD Inv POM.

Let the amount of morphine hydrochloride be x. Setting up proportional sets:

	amount (g)	molecular weight
morphine hydrochloride	x	376
morphine anhydrous base	0.4	285

$$\frac{x}{0.4} = \frac{376}{285}$$

$$x = 0.528$$

0.528 g of morphine hydrochloride is equivalent to 0.4 g of anhydrous morphine base. The maximum amount of morphine hydrochloride that can be incorporated into 200 mL of a liquid preparation so that the legal classification is CD Inv POM is 0.528 g.

Classification based on maximum strength and maximum dose

Some legal classifications are based on a maximum strength and a maximum dose, for example codeine. Codeine is CD POM but 'if for non-parenteral use and (a) in undivided preparations with ms 2.5% (calculated as base) CD Inv POM; or (b) in single dose preparations with ms per dosage unit 100 mg (calculated as base) CD Inv POM'.

Example 10.13

What is the maximum amount of codeine phosphate that can be incorporated into 100 mL of syrup and into a dosage unit so that it is CD Inv POM?

codeine base has a molecular weight of 317 g

codeine phosphate has a molecular weight of 406 g

In order that the syrup be CD Inv POM, the maximum strength is 2.5% of codeine base which is 2.5 g per 100 mL. So we need to calculate the amount of codeine phosphate equivalent to 2.5 g of codeine base.

Let the weight of codeine phosphate be x. Setting up proportional sets:

	amount (mg)	molecular weight
codeine phosphate	x	406
codeine base	2.5	317

$$\frac{x}{25} = \frac{406}{317}$$
$$x = 3.2$$

Therefore, the syrup contains up to 3.2 g in 100 mL and remains CD Inv POM.

In order for the unit dose to be CD Inv POM it must contain no more than 100 mg codeine base.

Let the weight of codeine phosphate be x. Setting up proportional sets:

	amount (mg)	molecular weight
codeine phosphate	x	406
codeine base	100	317

$$\frac{x}{100} = \frac{406}{317}$$
$$x = \frac{406 \times 100}{317} = 128 \text{ mg}$$

So the single dose unit could contain 128 mg and below and be CD Inv POM; above this quantity it would be CD POM

Moles and millimoles

The atomic and molecular weights of a drug or excipient can be used as a method of defining an amount of a drug or excipient. In this method, the term 'mole' is used. The mole is the SI base unit for the amount of a substance. The substance can be atoms, molecules or ions and the mole is the atomic, molecular or ionic weight expressed in grams. For example, the atomic weight of iron is 56 and so 1 mole of iron weighs 56 g. Similarly, the molecular weight of sodium chloride is 58.5, therefore a mole of sodium chloride weighs 58.5 g and 2 moles of sodium chloride weigh $58.5 \times 2 = 117$ g.

However, a molecule of sodium chloride consists of one sodium ion and one chloride ion. As moles can refer to ions as well as molecules, it can be seen that one mole of sodium chloride contains one mole of sodium and one mole of chloride, therefore:

1 mole of sodium chloride weighs 58.5 g

1 mole of sodium ion weighs 23 g

1 mole of chloride ion weighs 35.5 g

Now consider ferrous sulfate, $FeSO_4.7H_2O$. The molecular weight is 278 and so 1 mole weighs 278 g. However, from the molecular formula and knowledge of the atomic weights it can be seen that ferrous sulfate contains:

1 mole of $Fe = 56$ g

1 mole of $S = 32$ g

4 moles of O, each mole of $O = 16$ g

7 moles of H_2O, each mole of water $= 18$ g.

In the same way that the system of weights and volumes has multiples and subdivisions (milli, micro, nano, etc.), so the mole has similar subdivisions and multiples:

1 mole contains 1000 millimoles (mmol)

1 millimole contains 1000 micromoles

1 micromole contains 1000 nanomoles

1 nanomole contains 1000 picomoles

Again we can use a place value approach:

moles – – millimoles – – micromoles – – nanomoles

Using these column headings it can be seen that 2 millimoles is equivalent to 0.002 moles or 2000 micromoles or 2 000 000 nanomoles:

moles – – millimoles – – micromoles – – nanomoles

      2   0 0 0   0 0 0

Similarly, 15 micromoles is equivalent to 0.015 millimoles or 15 000 nanomoles:

Millimoles – – micromoles – – nanomoles

      1 5   0 0 0

As moles are relatively large quantities (e.g. 1 mole of clindamycin is 425 g), the subdivisions of the mole are frequently used for pharmaceuticals.

The quantities of many drugs, especially electrolytes, are expressed in moles or their subdivisions.

Example 10.14

How many millimoles each of Na^+ and HCO_3^- are there in a 500-mg sodium bicarbonate capsule?

First, it is necessary to consider the molecular formula of sodium bicarbonate. Sodium bicarbonate consists of one ion of sodium and one ion of bicarbonate:

$NaHCO_3 = Na^+ + HCO_3^-$

1 mole of sodium bicarbonate weighs 84 g and contains 1 mole of sodium and 1 mole of bicarbonate ion.

The relationship between mass of drug and number of moles is proportional, so for sodium bicarbonate capsules each weighing 500 mg, let the number of moles be y. (Remember to keep the units of weight the same, i.e. if the molecular weight is in grams then the weight of

→

the drug should be in grams [500 mg $=$ 0.5 g].) Setting up proportional sets:

number of moles	y	1
amount of sodium bicarbonate (g)	0.5	84

$$y = \frac{0.5}{84}$$

$$y = 0.0059$$

A sodium bicarbonate capsule will contain 0.0059 mole (5.9 millimoles) of sodium bicarbonate. As 1 mole of sodium bicarbonate consists of 1 mole of sodium and 1 mole of bicarbonate, 5.9 millimoles of sodium bicarbonate will contain 5.9 millimoles of sodium and 5.9 millimoles of bicarbonate ion.

If a molecule contains more than one ion of the same species, then care must be taken in calculating the number of moles.

Example 10.15

Calculate the number of moles of chloride ion in 500 mg of calcium chloride.

1 mole of calcium chloride ($CaCl_2$) consists of 1 mole of calcium and 2 moles of chloride ion. In order to calculate the number of moles of chloride ion in 500 mg of calcium chloride, it is necessary to calculate the number of moles of calcium chloride.

Let the number of moles of calcium chloride be z. The molecular weight of calcium chloride is 110. (Remember to keep the weights in the same units, i.e. convert 500 mg to 0.5 g.) Setting up proportional sets:

number of moles	z	1
amount of calcium chloride (g)	0.5	110

$$z = \frac{0.5}{110}$$

$$z = 0.0045$$

(continued)

The number of moles of calcium chloride is $0.0045 = 4.5$ millimoles, so 500 mg calcium chloride contains 4.5 millimoles of calcium chloride. It also contains 4.5 millimoles of calcium and 9.0 millimoles (4.5×2) of chloride ions, because there are twice as many chloride ions as calcium ions in calcium chloride.

If a salt contains water of crystallisation, then this should be taken into account when calculating moles. For example, a hydrated form of calcium chloride is $CaCl_2.6H_2O$. A mole of this hydrated form of calcium chloride will contain 1 mole of calcium ion, 2 moles of chloride ion and 6 moles of water.

Example 10.16

Using the above information, calculate the number of moles of water in 500 mg of $CaCl_2.6H_2O$.

The molecular weight of this molecule is 219 and it contains 6 moles of water. The number of moles of water in 500 mg (0.5 g) of hydrated calcium chloride can be calculated.

Let the number of moles of water be y. Setting up proportional sets:

| number of moles of water | y | 6 |
| amount of hydrated calcium chloride (g) | 0.5 | 219 |

$$\frac{y}{0.5} = \frac{6}{219}$$
$$y = 0.0137$$

There is 0.0137 mole of water $= 13.7$ millimoles.

Molar solutions

As a mole of a substance is defined as a weight, moles are one way of expressing a quantity or an amount. If 1 mole of a substance is dissolved in a solvent and the resulting solution made up to 1 L, then we have 1 mole in 1 L, which is an expression of concentration. This concentration can also be written as $1\,mol/L$ or $1\,mol\,L^{-1}$. Traditionally, the concentration of 1 mole per litre was called a molar solution.

For example, a $1\,mol/L$ aqueous solution of sodium chloride is equivalent to $58.5\,g$ of sodium chloride dissolved in sufficient water to produce $1\,L$ of solution. In other words, molarity refers to the number of moles of solute per litre of solution. As the term 'molar' is a concentration, it is not necessary to always prepare $1\,L$ of the solution; smaller volumes can be prepared.

Example 10.17

How many moles of solute are there in 20 mL of a 1 mol/L solution?

Let the number of moles of solute be y. Setting up proportional sets:

number of moles	y	1
volume of molar solution (mL)	20	1000

$$y = \frac{20}{1000}$$
$$y = 0.02$$

There is 0.02 mole of solute in 200 mL of a 1 mol/L solution.

It may be necessary to calculate the mass of a drug required to prepare a solution expressed in molar terms.

Example 10.18

How much sodium chloride is required to make 25 mL of a 0.5 molar solution? How many moles of sodium ion will there be in the final solution?

First it is necessary to find the molecular weights of sodium and sodium chloride and calculate how many moles of each are contained in 25 mL. The molecular weight of sodium is $23\,g$ and that of sodium chloride is $58.5\,g$.

(continued)

Let the number of moles of sodium chloride in 25 mL be y. Setting up proportional sets:

number of moles	y	0.5
volume of solution (mL)	25	1000

$$\frac{y}{25} = \frac{0.5}{1000}$$
$$y = 0.0125$$

There is 0.0125 mole of sodium chloride in 25 mL.

The mass of sodium chloride that is contained in 0.0125 mole of sodium chloride is obtained from the number of moles (0.0125) times the molecular weight of sodium chloride, i.e. 0.73125 g of sodium chloride; 0.73 g of sodium chloride would therefore be required to make 25 mL of a 0.5 molar solution. However, we know that 1 mole of sodium chloride contains 1 mole of sodium ions, so the solution of sodium chloride will contain the same number of moles of sodium chloride as sodium, i.e. 25 mL of a 0.5 molar solution of sodium chloride will contain 0.0125 mole of sodium ions.

As the molecular weights of many drugs are large, e.g. the molecular weights of cortisone, glibenclamide and nifedipine are 402, 494 and 346, respectively, solubility constraints make it impossible to prepare 1 molar solutions. Also, in many instances molar concentrations of drugs are above the required therapeutic level, so such drugs are prepared in concentrations such as millimoles/L, millimoles/mL or even picomoles/mL.

Example 10.19

How many millimoles of sodium and chloride ions are contained in 1 L of Sodium Chloride Infusion BP? Sodium Chloride Infusion BP contains 0.9% sodium chloride.

We know from Example 10.18 that 1 mole of sodium chloride contains 1 mole of sodium ions and 1 mole of chloride ions and that the weight of 1 mole of sodium chloride is 58.5 g. We can also calculate that there are 9 g of sodium chloride in 1 L of 0.9% sodium chloride.

→

Let the number of moles of sodium chloride in 1 L be x. Setting up proportional sets:

number of moles x 1

mass of sodium chloride (g)   9   58.5

$$x = \frac{9}{58.5}$$

$$x = 0.154$$

There is 0.154 mole of sodium chloride in 1 L of Sodium Chloride Infusion BP, so there is also 0.154 mole of sodium ions and 0.154 mole of chloride ions in the Infusion. Using the place value approach, it can be seen that 0.154 mole is equal to 154 millimoles. Thus Sodium Chloride Infusion BP contains 154 millimoles/L of sodium ions and chloride ions.

Some infusion fluids may contain more than one electrolyte, e.g. Potassium Chloride and Sodium Chloride Infusion Fluid BP. In such fluids the chloride ion concentration will be the sum of the chloride ion concentrations of both the potassium and the sodium salts.

Example 10.20

How many millimoles/L of chloride ions are contained in Potassium Chloride and Sodium Chloride Infusion BP?

The infusion fluid contains:

potassium chloride 0.3%   (3 g in 1 L)

sodium chloride 0.9%   (9 g in 1 L)

We know from the chemical formulae that 1 mole of both potassium chloride and sodium chloride would each contain 1 mole of chloride ions, so in order to calculate the number of moles of chloride ions in the infusion, we need to calculate the number of moles of both the potassium chloride and the sodium chloride. The molecular weights of sodium chloride and potassium chloride are, respectively, 58.5 and 74.5. The number of moles per litre of sodium chloride is calculated in Example 10.19 to be 154 millimoles, so we need to calculate the number of moles of potassium chloride by the same method.

(continued)

Let the number of moles of potassium chloride in 1 L be x. Setting up proportional sets:

number of moles of potassium chloride	x	1
amount of potassium chloride (g)	3	74.5

$$x = \frac{3}{74.5}$$

$$x = 0.04$$

There is 0.04 mole of potassium chloride in 1 L. The sodium chloride will contribute 0.154 mole of chloride ions to the infusion fluid and the potassium chloride will contribute 0.04 mole of chloride ions. This is a total of 0.194 mole of chloride ions. Converting moles to millimoles will give 194 millimoles of chloride ions in 1 L of infusion fluid.

From the above it can be seen that Potassium Chloride and Sodium Chloride Infusion BP will contain 154 millimoles of sodium ions and 40 millimoles of potassium ions per litre.

Example 10.21 involves calculating the mass of a drug required to prepare a known volume of a solution expressed in moles per litre.

Example 10.21

How much sodium fluoride will be required to make 250 mL of a mouthwash containing 0.012 mol/L of sodium fluoride?

The molecular weight of sodium fluoride is 42, so a 1 mol/L solution will contain 42 g in 1 L.

Let the number of grams of sodium fluoride in 0.012 mole be x. Setting up proportional sets:

number of moles	0.012	1
amount of sodium fluoride (g)	x	42

$$x = 42 \times 0.012$$

$$x = 0.504$$

$\rightarrow$

0.504 g of sodium fluoride is required to make 1 L of 0.012 mol/L mouthwash.

Let the quantity of sodium fluoride required to make 250 mL of mouthwash be y. Setting up proportional sets:

amount of sodium fluoride (g)	y	0.504
volume of mouthwash (mL)	250	1000

$$\frac{y}{250} = \frac{0.504}{1000}$$

$$y = 0.126$$

0.126 g of sodium fluoride is required to make 250 mL of mouthwash.

Moles

Practice calculations

Answers are given at the end of the chapter.

Q1   For the following drugs calculate the molecular weight and the weight of salt containing 1 millimole of the metal ion:

(a)   potassium chloride, KCl

(b)   sodium chloride, NaCl

(c)   calcium chloride, $CaCl_2.2H_2O$

(d)   calcium lactate, $C_6H_{10}CaO_6.5H_2O$

(e)   potassium bicarbonate, $KHCO_3$

(f)   magnesium chloride, $MgCl_2.6H_2O$

(g)   sodium citrate, $C_6H_5Na_3O_7.2H_2O$

(h)   ammonium chloride, NH_4Cl

Q2   (a)   Calculate the molecular weight of lithium citrate $(C_6H_5Li_3O_7.H_2O)$.

(b)   What is the percentage of Li^+ in lithium citrate?

Q3   (a)   The empirical formula of ferrous fumarate is $C_4H_2FeO_4$. Calculate its molecular weight.

(b)   Calculate the weight of ferrous fumarate that will give 100 mg of iron.

Q4   A syrup contains ferrous fumarate 140 mg/5 mL. How much iron will a patient receive per day if the daily dosage regimen is 10 mL twice a day?

Q5   A syrup contains 7.5% of potassium chloride. How many millimoles of K^+ are contained in 1 mL of this syrup?

Q6   Glucose intravenous infusion contains 5% glucose expressed as anhydrous glucose:

(a)   How much anhydrous glucose (molecular weight = 180) will be required to prepare 500 mL?

(b)   How much glucose monohydrate (molecular weight = 192) will be required to produce 750 mL of the infusion?

Q7   Calcium gluconate (molecular weight 448.4) tablets each contain 53.4 mg of calcium:

(a)   How much calcium gluconate does each tablet contain?

(b)   How many millimoles of calcium are there in each tablet?

Q8   (a)   What is the molecular weight of calcium acetate ($C_4H_6CaO_4$)?

(b)   Calculate the amount of calcium provided by 300 mg of calcium acetate.

(c)   How many milligrams of calcium acetate are there in 1 millimole?

Q9   (a)   What is the molecular weight of calcium phosphate ($Ca_3(PO_4)_2$)?

(b)   A powder contains 3.3 g of calcium phosphate. How many millimoles of calcium ion are provided by each powder?

Q10   Magnesium sulfate injection is 50% magnesium sulfate ($MgSO_4.7H_2O$). How many millimoles of magnesium ion per millilitre does the injection contain?

Q11   Sodium Fluoride BP drops contain 275 micrograms of sodium fluoride per drop. Calculate the quantity of fluoride ion provided by five drops of this preparation.

Q12 Ranitidine Injection BP contains ranitidine 25 mg/mL (as the hydrochloride). Calculate the amount of ranitidine hydrochloride needed to prepare 100 mL of injection. (Molecular weights: ranitidine hydrochloride = 350.9, ranitidine = 314.4.)

Q13 The term 'low sodium' indicates a sodium content of less than 1 millimole per tablet or 10-mL dose. What is the maximum amount of sodium chloride that can be contained in a 10-mL dose in order that the preparation can be labelled as 'low sodium'?

Q14 A syrup contains chloroquine sulfate (molecular weight = 436), 68 mg/5-mL dose. Calculate the amount of chloroquine base (molecular weight = 319.9) in each 5-mL dose.

Q15 How much chloroquine base (molecular weight = 319.9) is equivalent to a tablet containing 250 mg chloroquine phosphate (molecular weight = 515.9)?

Q16 How much morphine (molecular weight = 285.3) is contained in 50 mL of a 2% solution of morphine tartrate (molecular weight = 774.8)?

Q17 A patient requires 300 mg of quinine (molecular weight = 324.4). What weight of quinine hydrobromide (molecular weight = 423.3) will provide 300 mg of quinine?

Q18 How much hyoscine (molecular weight = 303.4) is contained in a 20-mg tablet of hyoscine butylbromide (molecular weight = 440.4)?

Answers

A1

	Molecular weight	Weight of 1 millimole (mg)
(a) potassium chloride, KCl	74.5	74.5
(b) sodium chloride, NaCl	58.5	58.5
(c) calcium chloride, $CaCl_2.2H_2O$	147	147
(d) calcium lactate, $C_6H_{10}CaO_6.5H_2O$	308	308
(e) potassium bicarbonate, $KHCO_3$	100	100
(f) magnesium chloride, $MgCl_2.6H_2O$	203	203
(g) sodium citrate, $C_6H_5Na_3O_7.2H_2O$	294.1	294.1
(h) ammonium chloride, NH_4Cl	53.5	53.5

A2 (a) 228
(b) 9.21%

A3 (a) 169.9
(b) 304 mg

A4 184 mg

A5 1 millimole

A6 (a) 25 g
(b) 40 g

A7 (a) 597.4 mg
(b) 1.33 millimoles

A8 (a) 158
(b) 75.9 mg
(c) 158 mg

A9 (a) 310
(b) 32 millimoles

A10 2 millimoles/mL

A11 622 micrograms

A12 2.79 g

A13 58.5 mg

A14 49.9 mg

A15 155 mg

A16 0.368 g

A17 391.5 mg

A18 13.8 mg

11

Parenteral solutions and isotonicity

Learning objectives

By the end of this chapter you will be able to:

- calculate the flow rate and amount of intravenous solution required for a patient
- calculate the volume of an intravenous solution that will deliver the correct amount of drug at the correct rate
- define the term 'isotonic' and calculate to produce isotonic solutions

The intravenous (IV) route, when a drug is introduced directly into a vein, is a common method for patients to receive drug therapy. The IV route involves the drug being presented as a sterile aqueous solution. If the volume to be delivered is a few millilitres or less, the solution (normally termed 'an injection') is usually administered in one go. If the volume to be delivered is large, it will be administered over a period of time. Such a process is termed 'intravenous infusion'. In order to deliver an IV infusion at a constant rate, a 'giving' or administration device consisting of an electrically driven pump will be used. The administration pump will be set to deliver a chosen number of drops or millilitres (mL) per minute or other unit of time.

With IV infusions, it may be necessary to calculate the volume of solution that is delivered over a period of time or the volume of solution that will deliver a known quantity of drug.

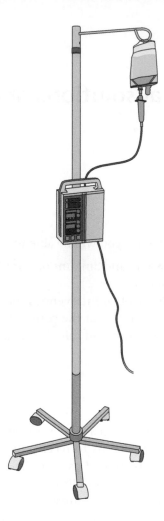

Rate of flow of intravenous solutions

Volume delivered over a specific time period

Calculations involving IV infusions may require the determination of the volume of drug solution delivered per period of time. This volume may be expressed as millilitres per minute or hour or the volume converted to drops per minute.

Example 11.1

One litre of 0.9% saline solution is to be given to a patient over a 6-hour period. If 20 drops = 1 mL, how many drops per minute should be administered?

The answer needs to be in minutes, so 6 hours is converted to 360 minutes.

The next stage involves calculating the number of drops in 1 litre, i.e. 1000 mL.

Let the number of drops be x. Setting up proportional sets:

number of drops	x	20
volume of solution (mL)	1000	1

$$\frac{x}{1000} = \frac{20}{1}$$
$$x = 20\,000$$

Therefore, there will be 20 000 drops in 1000 mL.

The infusion (of 20 000 drops) should take 360 minutes to complete. Let the number of drops per minute be y. Setting up proportional sets:

number of drops	20 000	y
number of minutes	360	1

$$\frac{y}{1} = \frac{20\,000}{360}$$
$$y = 55.5$$

Round up 55.5 to 56

Therefore, the IV administration set should be set for 56 drops per minute.

For some IV solutions a recommended flow rate is given. In which case, it may be necessary to calculate the overall volume to be delivered and the drops per minute.

Example 11.2

The recommended flow rate for drug Y is 2–3 mL/minute at a concentration of 5 mg/mL. Drug Y is supplied in 500-mg vials for dilution in glucose 5%. Using one vial of drug Y, what volume of glucose 5% solution should be used and how many drops per minute should be delivered if the flow rate is 3 mL/minute? The IV administration set is calibrated to 20 drops/mL. How long will the infusion take?

It is necessary to calculate the volume of glucose 5% required to produce a solution containing 5 mg of drug Y per mL. A vial of drug Y contains 500 mg.

Let the volume of solution required to contain 5 mg/mL be y mL. Setting up proportional sets:

drug Y (mg)	5	500
volume of solution (mL)	1	y

$$\frac{y}{500} = \frac{1}{5}$$
$$y = 100$$

Therefore, the vial of drug Y should be dissolved in sufficient glucose 5% to produce 100 mL of solution.

Knowing that the IV administration set produces 20 drops/mL, the number of drops in 3 mL can be calculated. Let the number of drops be x. Setting up proportional sets:

number of drops	x	20
volume (mL)	3	1

$$x = 60$$

3 mL is delivered in 1 minute so the IV infusion set should give a flow rate of 60 drops per minute.

$\rightarrow$

Let the time taken to administer 100 mL of infusion solution be t minutes. Setting up proportional sets:

time (minutes)	t	1
volume (mL)	100	3

$t = 33.3$

Therefore, the time taken to deliver 100 mL is 33.3 minutes.

In some situations, two or more injection solutions may be combined and delivered by IV infusion over a known time period. In such cases it is important to remember that the total volume of all the injection solutions should be included in the calculation.

Example 11.3

20 mL of Addiphos solution and 10 mL of multivitamin infusion are added to 500 mL of glucose 5% solution. The resultant solution is to be administered over 4 hours. The administration set is calibrated to 20 drops/mL. Calculate the number of drops per minute to be given if the patient is to receive all of the solution in the specified time.

The total volume of the infusion solution is:

20 mL + 10 mL + 500 mL = 530 mL

Therefore, 530 mL of solution must be infused over 4 hours.

As we need to calculate the number of drops per minute, we will need to convert the total infusion time to minutes:

total infusion time = 4 × 60 = 240 minutes

(*continued*)

The administration set gives 20 drops/mL and so we need to convert the total infusion volume into drops. Let the number of drops be x. Setting up proportional sets:

number of drops	20	x
volume (mL)	1	530

$x = 10\,600$

Therefore, 530 mL is equal to 10 600 drops.

10 600 drops of infusion solution will need to be delivered over 240 minutes.

Let the drops per minute required to deliver the infusion solution be y. Setting up proportional sets:

number of drops	y	10 600
time (minutes)	1	240

$$y = \frac{10\,600}{240}$$

$y = 44.17$

Therefore, the infusion fluid should be infused at 44 drops per minute.

Amount of drug delivered over a specified time period

With some drugs, the IV administration is stated as the amount of drug, rather than the volume, to be infused over a specified time period.

Example 11.4

A 56-kg female patient requires amphotericin by IV infusion at a dose of 250 micrograms/kg. The concentration of the final solution must not be more than 100 micrograms/mL. A vial of amphotericin contains 50 mg. Calculate the dose of amphotericin and the volume of IV solution required by the patient if the solution contains the maximum concentration. If the solution has to be delivered in 2.5 hours, what is the rate in mL/minute?

→

If a 50-mg vial is used to prepare the IV solution, what is the total volume of the solution prepared?

First the dose should be calculated.

Let the dose required be x. Setting up proportional sets:

amount of drug (micrograms)	250	x
body weight (kg)	1	56

$x = 250 \times 56$

$x = 14\,000$ micrograms

The patient requires a dose of 14 000 micrograms of amphotericin.

If the maximum concentration of amphotericin is 100 micrograms/mL, then the volume required for 14 000 micrograms will need to be calculated.

Let the volume required be z. Setting up proportional sets:

volume (mL)	1	z
amount of drug (micrograms)	100	14 000

$z = \dfrac{14\,000}{100}$

$z = 140$

Therefore, the patient will need 140 mL of infusion fluid containing 14 000 micrograms of drug.

If the infusion has to be over 2.5 hours, then the rate of delivery must be calculated. Let the rate of delivery per minute be y. Setting up proportional sets and converting 2.5 hours to 150 minutes:

volume (mL)	140	y
delivery time (minutes)	150	1

$y = \dfrac{140}{150}$

$y = 0.93$

The delivery rate will be 0.93 mL/minute.

(continued)

Amphotericin is available in a vial containing 50 mg. The total volume to contain the amphotericin at a concentration of 100 micrograms/mL needs to be calculated.

Let the total volume be v and convert 50 mg to 50 000 micrograms. Setting up proportional sets:

volume (mL)	1	v
drug (micrograms)	100	50 000

$$v = \frac{50\,000}{100}$$

$$v = 500$$

Therefore, the 50 mg of amphotericin needs to be dissolved in up to 500 mL of solvent, but only 140 mL will be administered to the patient.

The following example requires the infusion volume to be calculated.

Example 11.5

Phenytoin has a recommended dose of 18 mg/kg of body weight to be infused at a rate not exceeding 50 mg/minute. Assume that the patient is a woman weighing 56 kg. Phenytoin injection is available in 5-mL ampoules containing 50 mg/mL. The prescriber would like an infusion volume of 100 mL and a dose rate of 25 mg/minute. Is the prescriber's request possible and, if so, what is the flow rate per minute?

It is necessary to calculate the recommended dose for the patient.
    The patient weighs 56 kg and the dose is 18 mg/kg.
    Let the required dose be z. Setting up proportional sets:

dose (mg)	18	z
weight (kg)	1	56

$$z = 18 \times 56$$

$$z = 900$$

Therefore, the recommended dose for the patient is 900 mg phenytoin.
    The injection contains 50 mg/mL.

$\rightarrow$

Let the volume of injection (mL) be *y*. Setting up proportional sets:

| phenytoin (mg) | 900 | 50 |
| volume of injection (mL) | *y* | 1 |

$$y = \frac{900}{50}$$
$$y = 18$$

Therefore, 18 mL of phenytoin injection is required for the recommended dose.

Clearly this volume could be made up to 100 mL with 0.9% saline solution as requested by the prescriber. The resulting 100 mL of solution will contain 900 mg of phenytoin. It is now necessary to calculate the volume per minute that will be needed to deliver 25 mg/minute. In other words, the volume that contains 25 mg of phenytoin.

Let the volume required in mL be *x*. Setting up proportional sets:

| phenytoin (mg) | 900 | 25 |
| volume of solution (mL) | 100 | *x* |

$$\frac{x}{25} = \frac{100}{900}$$
$$x = 2.78$$

Therefore, 2.78 mL contains 25 mg of phenytoin. Thus the flow rate of the infusion should be set at 2.78 mL/minute.

Some drugs will be given in much smaller injection volumes through a micropump device. This device enables very small volumes to be delivered at a set rate for a specified time period.

Example 11.6

The required dose of furosemide by slow IV infusion is 50 mg at a rate not exceeding 4 mg/minute. Furosemide injection contains 10 mg furosemide in 1 mL. Calculate the volume of furosemide injection required and the infusion rate, i.e. mL/minute, if the patient is to receive the correct dose.

(continued)

First calculate the volume of injection required.

The injection is available as 10 mg/mL and a total of 50 mg is required.

Let the required volume of injection in mL be y. Setting up proportional sets:

volume of injection (mL)	1	y
mass of furosemide (mg)	10	50

$$y = \frac{50}{10}$$

$$y = 5$$

Therefore, 5 mL of injection is required and this must be given at a maximum rate of 4 mg/minute. Knowing this maximum rate, we need to calculate the time to deliver 50 mg of furosemide at this rate.

Let the time to deliver 50 mg of furosemide in minutes be z. Setting up proportional sets:

furosemide (mg)	4	50
time (minutes)	1	z

We can spot that 4 is divided by 4 to give 1, so 50 is divided by 4 to give z

$$z = 12.5$$

Therefore, it will take 12.5 minutes to deliver all the injection solution at 4 mg/minute.

Let the volume to be delivered in one minute be x. Setting up proportional sets:

volume (mL)	5	x
time (minutes)	12.5	1

$$\frac{x}{1} = \frac{5}{12.5}$$

$$x = 0.4$$

Therefore, the infusion device should be set at a maximum of 0.4 mL/minute.

If a drug is to be administered over a long time period, e.g. 12 hours or more, then the flow rate may be expressed in mg/hour rather than mg/minute. In such a case, care must be taken not to confuse minutes with hours, otherwise the dose will be wrong and the treatment of the patient compromised.

Example 11.7

A drug is provided as an infusion solution at a concentration of 0.15 mg/mL. The prescribed flow rate is 3 mg/hour. Calculate the flow rate in mL/minute and drops/minute if 1 mL = 20 drops.

The answer is required in minutes, so it is necessary to convert the flow rate of mg/hour to rate in mg/minute.

Let the number of mg per minute be y. Setting up proportional sets:

drug (mg)	3	y
time (minutes)	60	1

$$y = \frac{3}{60}$$
$$y = 0.05$$

Therefore, the flow rate is 0.05 mg/minute.

Now we need to find the volume of solution that contains 0.05 mg. We know that the solution contains 0.15 mg/mL.

Let the volume of solution (in mL) that contains 0.05 mg be x. Setting up proportional sets:

volume of solution (mL)	1	x
drug (mg)	0.15	0.05

$$x = \frac{0.05}{0.15}$$
$$x = 0.33$$

Therefore, 0.33 mL of solution contains 0.05 mg of drug. As the drug has to be given at the rate of 0.05 mg/minute, the correct flow rate for the drug solution will be 0.33 mL/minute.

(continued)

Given that 1 mL is equivalent to 20 drops, it is possible to convert 0.33 mL to drops. Let the number of drops in 0.33 mL be z. Setting up proportional sets:

number of drops	20	z
volume (mL)	1	0.33

$z = 20 \times 0.33$

$z = 6.7$

Therefore, the administration set should be adjusted to give 7 drops/minute.

Some solutions of drugs are required to be delivered continuously and subcutaneously. In such a situation a syringe driver may be used. The syringe driver will be calibrated as the distance the driver moves per unit of time. Therefore, it is necessary to calculate the rate of delivery in order to give a known amount of drug.

Example 11.8

Apomorphine injection may be given via a syringe driver with a rate setting in mm/hour. Apomorphine injection contains 10 mg/mL. It is usual to dilute the injection with an equal volume of sodium chloride 0.9% before adding to the 10-mL syringe. The 10-mL syringe has a length of 60 mm. If the patient requires 2.5 mg of apomorphine per hour, at what rate setting should the syringe driver be fixed?

First it is necessary to calculate the amount of drug contained in the 10-mL syringe.

The apomorphine solution is prepared by mixing 5 mL of apomorphine injection with 5 mL of sodium chloride solution; 5 mL of apomorphine injection (10 mg/mL) contains 50 mg of apomorphine and so there must be 50 mg of apomorphine in the 10 mL of solution.

→

The patient requires 2.5 mg of apomorphine per hour and we know that 50 mg is contained in 10 mL. We also know that the 10 mL is contained in a syringe that is 60 mm in length. Therefore, we need to calculate the number of millimetres that will contain 2.5 mg.

Let the number of mm containing 2.5 mg be x. Setting up proportional sets:

length (mm)	60	x
apomorphine (mg)	50	2.5

$$\frac{x}{2.5} = \frac{60}{50}$$
$$x = \frac{60 \times 2.5}{50}$$
$$x = 3$$

Therefore, 3 mm of the syringe contains 2.5 mg of apomorphine. If the patient is to receive 2.5 mg/hour, the syringe driver should be set at 3 mm/hour.

In some situations, a syringe driver may be set to one rate of delivery and so the concentration of drug in the syringe has to be calculated as in the following example.

Example 11.9

A 100-mg dose of an analgesic has to be infused over a 5-hour period. The drug is available in 1-mL vials each containing 50 mg of the drug. The only syringe driver available has a 20-mL capacity syringe, which delivers at a constant rate of 2 mL/hour. How many vials of the drug and what volume of diluent will be required to fill the 20-mL syringe so that the drug is delivered at the correct concentration? (The syringe driver can be set to automatically stop after 5 hours.)

First we need to calculate the amount of drug required per hour.

(continued)

Let the amount (mg) of drug per hour be x. Setting up proportional sets:

amount of drug (mg)	100	x
time (hours)	5	1

$$x = \frac{100}{5}$$
$$x = 20$$

The patient requires 20 mg of drug per hour.

If the rate of delivery is 2 mL/hour, then 2 mL of the drug solution will need to contain 20 mg. The capacity of the syringe driver is 20 mL, so we need to calculate the total amount of drug to be contained in 20 mL. Let the amount of drug in 20 mL be y. Setting up proportional sets:

amount of drug (mg)	20	y
volume of solution (mL)	2	20

$$y = 200 \text{ mg}$$

Therefore, the 20-mL syringe driver will need to contain 200 mg of analgesic drug. The drug is available as 1-mL vials each containing 50 mg.

Let the number of vials required be z. Setting up proportional sets:

number of vials	1	z
amount of drug (mg)	50	200

$$z = 4$$

Therefore, four vials each containing 50 mg will provide the required amount of drug.

The volume of diluent required to produce 20 mL of drug solution will be:

$$20 - 4 = 16 \text{ mL}$$

Isotonicity

Solutions of drugs that are placed in contact with mucous membranes may cause stinging, irritation and cell destruction. These effects can be minimised by making the solution isotonic with the mucous membrane.

Osmotic pressure is a property of ions or molecules dissolved in water. Similarly freezing point depression is related to the ions/molecules dissolved in water. It is the relationship between freezing point depression and osmotic pressure that is used in the formulation of isotonic and iso-osmotic solutions.

A 0.9% w/v solution of sodium chloride in water is iso-osmotic with blood, serum and other body fluids such as tears. In other words it has the same osmotic pressure; 0.9% w/v sodium chloride solution freezes at −0.52°C and so do blood, serum and other body fluids. Thus other solutions that freeze at −0.52°C will be isotonic with blood, serum, etc. A 0.9% w/v solution of sodium chloride is known as 'physiological saline solution', '0.9% saline solution' or 'a normal saline solution'.

A solution of a small amount of a drug in water will probably have an osmotic pressure less than that of body fluids. In order to make the solution isotonic, it is necessary to add another substance. The usual adjusting substance is sodium chloride, because it is found in body fluids and is non-toxic. A table of iso-osmotic concentrations and freezing point depressions for many drugs can be found in *The Pharmaceutical Codex*.

The proportional sets approach can be used to calculate the amount of adjusting substance required to add to a solution in order to make it isotonic.

However, the relationship between freezing point depression and concentration of the ion or molecule is not linear, although all methods of calculation assume a linear relationship over a small temperature range. So in practice all solutions should be tested for isotonicity to ensure that the theoretical calculations (whatever method is used) are valid.

Example 11.10

Calculate the amount of sodium chloride that should be added to the following formulation of nasal drops in order to make the final solution isotonic.

ephedrine hydrochloride	*0.5 g*
water to	*100 mL*

(continued)

(A 1% w/v solution of ephedrine hydrochloride depresses the freezing point by 0.169°C.
A 1% w/v solution of sodium chloride depresses the freezing point by 0.576°C.)

Remember: an isotonic solution freezes at −0.52°C.

It is necessary to calculate the freezing point depression attributable to the ephedrine hydrochloride.

Let the freezing point depression caused by the ephedrine be x. Setting up proportional sets:

ephedrine hydrochloride (% w/v)	1	0.5
freezing point depression (°C)	0.169	x

(*Note*: if the relationship between freezing point depression and percentage w/v concentration is not linear then the sets will not be proportional.)

$$\frac{x}{0.5} = \frac{0.169}{1}$$
$$x = 0.0845$$

Therefore, the ephedrine hydrochloride depresses the freezing point to 0.0845°C below 0°C, i.e. to −0.0845°C.

Thus the added sodium chloride will be required to depress the freezing point of the ephedrine solution, i.e. a further 0.4355°C so that it reaches the isotonic solution freezing point of −0.52°C.

The required amount of sodium chloride to be added to the ephedrine hydrochloride solution has to be calculated.

Let the freezing point depression caused by the added sodium chloride be z. Setting up proportional sets:

sodium chloride (% w/v)	1	z
freezing point depression (°C)	0.576	0.4355

$$\frac{z}{0.4355} = \frac{1}{0.576}$$
$$z = \frac{0.4355}{0.576}$$
$$z = 0.756$$

Therefore, 0.756% w/v of sodium chloride should be added to the formula to ensure that the final solution is isotonic.

Parenteral doses

Answers are given at the end of the chapter.

Q1   1 L of glucose 5% solution is to be given to a patient over a 5-hour period. Calculate the rate of delivery in mL/minute.

Q2   500 mL of 0.9% saline solution is to be given to a patient over a 6-hour period. If 20 drops = 1 mL, calculate how many drops per minute should be administered to the patient?

Q3   An IV solution is to be administered at a rate of 2 mL/minute. What volume will be required if the infusion is to be maintained for 3 hours?

Q4   A 10-mL vial of multivitamin injection is to be added to 500 mL of glucose 5% solution. The resultant solution is to be administered to a patient over 3 hours. The administration set is calibrated at 20 drops/mL. Calculate the number of drops per minute to be given if the patient is to receive all the solution in the specified time.

Q5   Nizatidine injection (25 mg/mL) is supplied in 4-mL vials. The BNF states that for continuous infusion 'dilute 300 mg in 150 mL and give at a rate of 10 mg/hour'. If this procedure is adopted, calculate:

   (a)   how many vials of nizatidine injection will be required

   (b)   the flow rate (in mL/hour)

   (c)   the length of time the infusion will take.

Q6   A pharmacist prepares a solution of vancomycin containing 1 g in 200 mL. The rate of infusion should not exceed 10 mg/minute.

   (a)   Calculate the maximum flow rate in mL/minute.

   (b)   If the decision is to give the infusion over 2 hours, calculate the flow rate in mL/minute.

Q7   A baby weighing 3.4 kg requires treatment with phenytoin at a dose of 20 mg/kg. A 5-mL vial of phenytoin injection containing 50 mg/mL is available for dilution before infusion. A suitable volume of phenytoin injection is diluted up to 50 mL with sodium chloride 0.9%.

   (a)   Calculate the volume of phenytoin injection that must be used in the preparation of the infusion.

(b) The infusion rate must not exceed 3 mg/kg/minute. Calculate the maximum flow rate in mL/minute if these conditions are applied to the administration.

(c) The infusion must be completed in 1 hour. Calculate the minimum flow rate (in mL/minute) if the infusion is completed in 1 hour.

Q8 The recommended dose of drug X is 75 mg by slow infusion at a rate not exceeding 0.3 g/hour. Drug X is available as an injection containing 15 mg of drug X in 1 mL. Calculate the volume of drug X injection required and the infusion rate in mL/minute.

Q9 A drug is provided as an infusion solution at a concentration of 2 micrograms/mL. The prescribed flow rate is 0.05 mg/hour. Calculate the flow rate in mL/minute and drops/minute if 1 mL = 25 drops.

Q10 A syringe driver is designed to contain 5 mL of injection and has a length of 60 mm. Injection Y contains 4 mg/mL. If a patient requires 2.5 mg of drug Y per hour, at what rate setting in mm/hour should the syringe driver be fixed?

Q11 A syringe driver is set at 5 mm/hour. The length of the syringe driver is 80 mm and it holds 10 mL of injection solution. An injection solution contains 5 micrograms of drug X in 1 mL. What dose of drug X will the syringe driver deliver in 3 hours?

Q12 An IV solution of sodium chloride 0.2% needs to be made isotonic by the addition of anhydrous glucose. What weight of anhydrous glucose is required in the preparation of 1 L of the IV solution? (A 1% solution of sodium chloride depresses the freezing point of water by 0.576°C. A 1% solution of anhydrous glucose depresses the freezing point of water by 0.1037°C.)

Q13 Zinc sulfate 0.25% eye drops are required to be made isotonic with sodium chloride. What weight of sodium chloride is required in the preparation of 100 mL of eye-drop solution? (A 0.25% solution of zinc sulfate depresses the freezing point of water by 0.022°C.)

Q14 How much sodium chloride should be added in the preparation of 25 mL of pilocarpine hydrochloride 2% eye drops to render them isotonic? (A 2% solution of pilocarpine hydrochloride depresses the freezing point of water by 0.262°C.)

Q15 Using the information in Question 14, explain why it may not be possible or necessary to make pilocarpine hydrochloride 4% eye drops isotonic.

Q16 How much sodium chloride is required in the preparation of 50 mL of isotonic amethocaine hydrochloride 0.5% solution? Assume the sodium chloride is used for isotonicity adjustment only. (A 0.5% solution of amethocaine hydrochloride depresses the freezing point of water by 0.062°C.)

Answers

A1   3.33 mL/minute

A2   28 drops/minute

A3   360 mL

A4   56.6 drops/minute

A5   (a) three vials
(b) 5 mL/hour
(c) 30 h

A6   (a) 2 mL/minute
(b) 1.66 mL/minute

A7   (a) 1.36 mL
(b) 7.5 mL/minute
(c) 0.833 mL/minute

A8   5 mL
0.33 mL/minute

A9   0.417 mL/minute
10.4 drops/minute

A10   7.5 mm/hour

A11   9.357 micrograms

A12   39.03 g

A13   0.864 g

A14   0.112 g

A15   The depression due to 4% pilocarpine hydrochloride is 0.524°C, which is about the same as that of an isotonic solution.

A16   0.398 g

12

Accuracy of measurement

Learning objectives

By the end of this chapter you will be able to:

- round a number and use rounding techniques in calculations
- correct a number to significant figures or places of decimals
- calculate limits for weights in pharmaceutical assays and tests
- calculate limits for the contents of pharmaceutical substances and their formulations

Consider the following statement:

> The dispensary is 15.342 metres long

In the 15.342 metres, the last figure, 2, is in the millimetres column and so the length of the dispensary in millimetres is 15 342. It is unlikely that anyone would want to know the length of the room to that degree of accuracy and it is also unlikely that the measurements could be made to that degree of accuracy without very specialised equipment. The figure 2 is likely to be unnecessary and may also be misleading, implying that the measurement is more accurate than it really is.

Sometimes we need to express numbers 'to the nearest'. For example, if we need the above dispensary length to the nearest centimetre, the result would be 1534 cm. Its length to the nearest metre would be 15 metres. This 'to the nearest' approach brings us to the technique of rounding.

Rounding numbers

Rounding is used to make numbers more convenient or smaller so that numbers are easier to work with, especially if you are trying to work the answers out in your head. However, rounded numbers are only approximate and so an exact answer, generally, cannot be obtained using rounded numbers.

In order to round a number we look, normally, at the last figure or figures:

If the number ends in 1 to 4, then the number is converted to the next lower number that ends in 0. For example, 54 rounded to the nearest 10 becomes 50.

If the number ends in 5 to 9, then the number is converted to the next higher number ending in 0. For example, 58 rounded to the nearest 10 becomes 60.

Rounded numbers are used to get an answer that is close to the exact answer, but is unlikely to be the exact number. For example, if we need to add together 199 and 2254, then by rounding each number to the nearest 10:

199 becomes 200 and

2254 becomes 2250

The total of the two rounded numbers is 2450 compared with the total of the unrounded numbers, which is 2453.

The technique of rounded numbers is used to reduce a number with several figures to one with fewer figures or to reduce a number with a large number of figures after the decimal place to a more convenient or manageable size.

Significant figures

Converting the dispensary length from nearest metres (15) to nearest centimetres gives a length of 1500 centimetres. In this number, the 1 means one thousand, the 5 means five hundreds, but the 00 does not mean 0 tens and 0 units. The 00 means that the number of tens and the number of units are not stated. The zeros are there to act as spacers so that the 1 appears in the thousands column and the 5 appears in the hundreds column. As the 1 and the 5 mean what they say, they are significant figures. The two zeros are not significant figures.

Example 12.1

A bottle contains 80 mL of a liquid to the nearest 10 mL. How many significant figures are there?

The 8 means 8 tens but the 0 means that the number of units is not stated. There is one significant figure.

Example 12.2

A bottle contains 0.04 L of a liquid to the nearest 0.01 L. How many significant figures are there?

The number 0.04 can be written as 0.040. The 0 to the right of the 4 means that the number of thousandths of a litre is unknown and it and any more zeros that may be written to the right of it are not significant. The 4 means 4 hundredths of a litre and is significant. The 0 to the left of the 4 appears only as a spacer to make the 4 appear in the hundredths column so it is not significant. There is one significant figure.

Example 12.3

The number 152 000 is stated to the nearest hundred. How many significant figures are there?

The 0 after the 2 means that there are no hundreds. The following 00 means that the number of tens and the number of units are not stated. There are four significant figures.

Note: if a number is stated in the form 0.340 (rather than 0.34) and we are not told to what degree of accuracy the number is stated, the zero to the right of the 4 would be interpreted as indicating that there are no thousandths and that the number was correct to the nearest thousandth. There would be three significant figures. This way of expressing numbers is used to convey the degree of precision required in weights and measurements (see later).

Correcting to fewer significant figures

In order to correct 33.62 to two significant figures, we consider the first three significant figures. Using the rounding technique, 33.62 corrected to two significant figures is 34.

Similarly, in order to correct 33.42 to two significant figures, we consider the first three significant figures. Using the rounding technique, 33.42 corrected to two significant figures is 33.

Examples 12.4–12.7

Example 12.4
Correct 17 586 to three significant figures.

Answer 17 600

Example 12.5
Correct 17 536 to three significant figures.

Answer 17 500

Example 12.6
Correct 0.000 3274 to two significant figures.

Answer 0.000 33

Example 12.7
Correct 0.000 3234 to two significant figures.

Answer 0.000 32

Correcting to a certain number of decimal places

The method used is similar to that described above to deal with correction to a certain number of significant figures and again involves the rounding technique.

Look at the figure in the column to the right of the last decimal place required. If the figure is 4 or less, it and any digits to the right of it are deleted. If the digit is a 5 or higher, the digit of the last decimal place is increased by 1 and any digits to the right are deleted.

Examples 12.8–12.11

Example 12.8
Correct 1.5654 to three decimal places.

Answer 1.565

Example 12.9
Correct 1.5655 to three decimal places.

Answer 1.566

→

Example 12.10
Correct 21.7234 to two decimal places.

Answer 21.72

Example 12.11
Correct 21.7258 to two decimal places.

Answer 21.73

Accuracy in arithmetic calculations

If all the values involved in a calculation are exact then it will be possible to calculate the exact value of the result. If, however, some of the values involved in a calculation are inexact and have been stated to a certain number of significant figures, a decision needs to be made as to how many figures of the result are likely to be significant.

If the arithmetic operations involve addition and/or subtraction, then the rule applied states that the result should be rounded to the precision of the least precise approximate number involved. For example, assume in the following calculation that all numbers have been rounded and so are approximate.

$$234.56 + 876.5 - 654.321$$

The apparent result is 456.739. This result is to three decimal places. However, if we look at the three original numbers, the least precise is 876.5 because it is expressed only to one decimal place. If we apply the rule, then the result should be expressed and rounded to one decimal place, i.e. 456.7.

If the arithmetic operations involve multiplication and/or division, the rule is to find the number in the calculation that has the least number of significant figures, and to round the result to that number of significant figures. For example, assume in the following calculation that all the numbers have been rounded and so are approximate.

$$(234.56 \times 876.5) \div 654.321$$

The apparent result using a calculator is 314.206 3911. If we look at the three original numbers, the one with the least number of significant figures is 876.5 with four significant figures. If we apply the rule the result should be expressed and rounded to four significant figures, 314.2.

However, be aware that the actual number of reliable significant figures could be even smaller. Throughout a calculation, numbers should be retained to more significant figures than those required in the final result and correcting to the required number of significant figures should be carried only out at the end of the calculation.

Errors built up in arithmetic calculations

When, because of measuring difficulties, numbers are stated as estimates to a certain number of significant figures, errors are introduced. Further errors are built up when calculations are carried out and, if there is a need to keep a close check on the extent of the errors, it is possible to do so by finding lower and upper bounds for the possible values of the result.

As an example of this approach, consider the expression:

$$\frac{21.3 \times 124.6}{32.4}$$

where each number is rounded and stated correct to one decimal place.

21.349 corrected to three significant figures becomes 21.3

21.312 corrected to three significant figures becomes 21.3

21.273 corrected to three significant figures becomes 21.3

21.251 corrected to three significant figures becomes 21.3

Thus, we can see that any number in the interval from 21.25 to 21.35 (but not including the number 21.35) will be represented by the number 21.3 after correction to three significant figures. So in using 21.3 there is a possible error of up to 0.09. Similarly, 124.6 represents any number in the interval from 124.55 to 124.65 and 32.4 represents any number in the interval from 32.35 to 32.45.

When 21.3 is multiplied by 124.6, the smallest value that can be obtained is the one achieved by multiplying the smallest value represented by 21.3 by the smallest value represented by 124.6, i.e. 21.25×124.55, giving 2646.6875. The smallest value of the result will be obtained by dividing 2646.6875 by the largest value represented by 32.4, i.e. 32.45, giving 81.562018.

When 21.3 is multiplied by 124.6, the largest value that can be obtained is the one achieved by multiplying the largest value represented by 21.3 by the largest value represented by 124.6, i.e. 21.35×124.65, giving 2661.2775. The largest value of the result will be obtained by dividing 2661.2775 by the smallest value represented by 32.4, i.e. 32.35, giving 82.265 147.

We have found lower and upper limits of 81.562 018 and 82.265 147 for the result of the calculation. Using a calculator to evaluate the expression, the result is 81.912 963. Each of these three values becomes 82 when corrected to two significant figures. Applying the rule stated above, values 21.3 and 32.4 are those involved in the calculation that have the least number of significant figures. Correcting the calculator result to the same number of significant figures gives 81.9, but we see that there is a possible error of about 0.35, so the third figure is in doubt. This supports the warning expressed earlier that the actual number of reliable significant figures may be smaller than that provided by the rule.

Accuracy in weighing/measuring for pharmaceutical tests and assays

The *European Pharmacopoeia* (EP) gives instructions for dealing with accuracy and precision. In tests and assays, the stated quantity to be taken is approximate, but the amount actually used is accurately weighed and the result is calculated from this exact quantity. In addition, the amount actually weighed may deviate by not more than 10% from that stated. The EP also gives instructions for quantities weighed or measured, which must have an accuracy commensurate with the indicated degree of precision. For example, in the case of weighing, the precision corresponds to plus or minus 5 units after the last figure stated, thus 0.25 g is to be interpreted as 0.245 g to 0.255 g. This is an example of rounding. The degree of precision is implied by the number of significant figures.

Use the following information to complete Examples 12.12, 12.13 and 12.14.

The EP states that erythromycin ethyl succinate should contain not more than 3.0% water determined on 0.300 g by semi-micro determination of water and not more than 0.3% of sulfated ash determined on 1.0 g.

Example 12.12

What are the limits on the weights of erythromycin used for the determination of water?

First let us consider the two weights, 0.300 g and 1.0 g. The precision of the required weighing is indicated by the number of significant figures:

0.300 g is three significant figures

1.0 g is two significant figures

In practice (because it would be extremely difficult to weigh an exact amount) the weight of a sample can vary by not more than 10%. These limits can be calculated using proportional sets. If 0.300 g represents 100% and the limits are set to 90% (10% less) and 110% (10% more), let x and y represent the unknown quantities for 90% and 110% respectively. Setting up proportional sets:

quantity (g)	0.300	x	y
percentage	100	90	110

$$x = \frac{0.300 \times 90}{100}$$

and

$$y = \frac{0.300 \times 110}{100}$$

$$x = 0.270$$

$$y = 0.330$$

Note: both these answers are expressed to the same number of significant figures as the original number.

Thus the actual weighing can be between 0.270 g and 0.330 g and must be recorded as the actual weight and not rounded.

Example 12.13

Assume that the operator weighed 0.2985 g of erythromycin ethyl succinate. What would be the maximum amount of water allowed in the sample expressed in grams?

→

Remember that the sample can contain not more than 3.0% of water.

Let 0.2985 g represent 100% and the unknown quantity of water equal x. Setting up proportional sets:

quantity (g)   0.2985 x

percentage   100   3.0

$$x = \frac{0.2985 \times 3.0}{100}$$

$x = 0.008955$

The sample can contain up to 0.008955 g of water, which rounded to three significant figures (the same number of significant figures as the weight of drug sample in the EP) is 0.009 g.

Example 12.14

An operator found that a 1.04 g sample of erythromycin ethyl succinate contained 0.0036 g of sulfated ash. Is this acceptable?

Remember that the sample can contain not more than 0.3% of sulfated ash.

Let 1.04 g represent 100% and the unknown quantity of sulfated ash be x. Setting up proportional sets:

quantity (g)   1.04 x

percentage   100   0.3

$$x = \frac{1.04 \times 0.3}{100}$$

$x = 0.00312$

Therefore, the sample can contain a maximum of 0.00312 g of sulfated ash in order to comply with the EP requirements. The sample was found to contain 0.0036 g of sulfated ash and so it will not comply.

Limits and uniformity of content

Some monographs in the EP express the content of a substance in terms of its chemical formula and in many cases the upper limit may exceed 100%. The limits are based on the results of the assay calculated in terms of the equivalent content of the specified chemical formula. For example, the EP monograph for aspirin (acetylsalicylic acid) states that it contains not less than 99.5% and not more than the equivalent of 101.0% of 2-acetoxybenzoic acid.

Similarly, because of production and manufacturing techniques, the EP states that aspirin tablets are required to contain aspirin, $C_9H_8O_4$, between 95.0% and 105.0% of the prescribed or stated amount. A similar statement is given for other tablets/capsules/dosage forms.

These limits can be calculated using proportional sets or using a calculator if you are competent at obtaining percentages.

Example 12.15

A 300-mg aspirin tablet is assayed for aspirin content. What are the EP limits for the aspirin content of this tablet?

Let 300 mg be equivalent to 100% and the unknown quantities representing 95% and 105% be x and y, respectively. Setting up proportional sets:

quantity of aspirin (mg)	300	x	y
Percentage	100	95.0	105.0

$$x = \frac{300 \times 95.0}{100}$$

$$y = \frac{300 \times 105.0}{100}$$

$$x = 285 \quad \text{and} \quad y = 315$$

Therefore, the aspirin tablet must contain between 285 mg and 315 mg if it is to comply with the monograph.

Answers are given at the end of the chapter.

Q1   The following are the published atomic weights for a number of elements. For each element state the number of significant figures, the number of places after the decimal point and convert each atomic weight to two and four significant figures.

Aluminium	26.9815
Barium	137.327
Boron	10.811
Hydrogen	1.0079
Platinum	195.08
Potassium	39.0983
Uranium	238.0289
Zinc	65.39

Q2   Atenolol oral solution contains 25 mg of atenolol per 5 mL. The EP states that the atenolol content should be 94% to 104% of the stated amount. If a patient takes 5 mL of atenolol solution every day for 28 days, calculate the total stated amount of atenolol. Compare this calculated amount with the total amount if the solution contained the lower limit of atenolol as stated in the EP.

Q3   Bupivacaine injection contains 2.5 mg of anhydrous bupivacaine hydrochloride per mL. The EP states that the content of anhydrous bupivacaine hydrochloride must be between 92.5% and 107.5% of the stated amount. A 10-mL vial of bupivacaine injection was assayed and found to contain 22.75 mg of anhydrous bupivacaine hydrochloride. Do the contents of this vial comply with the EP monograph and why?

Q4   Paediatric ferrous sulfate solution contains 12 g of ferrous sulfate in 1000 mL. The EP states that the content of ferrous sulfate in the solution is 1.10 to 1.30% w/v. If a child is given a 5-mL dose, calculate the upper limit of ferrous sulfate that would be in that dose, if the solution complied with the EP.

Q5 The following list gives the names of drugs and the limits imposed by the EP. For a 500-mg sample of each drug calculate the least equivalent amount that should be present (determined by assay) if the drug is to comply with the monograph.

Calculate the upper limit for each drug assuming the original sample size is 525 mg.

(a) mebendazole hydrochloride	98% to 101%
(b) methyltestosterone	97% to 103%
(c) pentobarbital sodium	99% to 101.5%
(d) amoxicillin sodium	85% to 100.5%
(e) cefotaxime sodium	96.0% to 101.0%

Q6 The EP's Uniformity of Content for transdermal patches states that the preparation complies with the test if the average content of ten dosage units is between 90% and 110% of the labelled content, and if the individual content of each dosage unit is between 75% and 125% of the average content. Assuming that each patch contains a stated 680 micrograms of norethisterone, calculate the upper and lower limits for the average content of ten patches. If the actual average for ten patches is 710 micrograms per patch, calculate the upper and lower limits for an individual patch.

Answers

A1

	Significant figures	After decimal point	Correct to two significant figures	Correct to four significant figures
Aluminium	6	4	27	26.98
Barium	6	3	140	137.3
Boron	5	3	11	10.81
Hydrogen	5	4	1.0	1.008
Platinum	5	2	200	195
Potassium	6	4	39	39.10
Uranium	7	4	240	238.0
Zinc	4	2	65	65.39

A2   700 mg; 658 mg

A3   No, the vial does not comply because the content is 91%.

A4   The upper limit would be 65 mg.

A5   (a) 490 mg; 530 mg
          (b) 485 mg; 541 mg
          (c) 495 mg; 533 mg
          (d) 425 mg; 528 mg
          (e) 480 mg; 530 mg

A6   6120 micrograms and 7480 micrograms; 533 micrograms and
          888 micrograms

13

Calculations involving information retrieval

Learning objectives

By the end of this chapter you will be able to:

- retrieve the correct information about a drug from an information source
- use retrieved information to perform a calculation
- determine the type of calculation that will produce the correct answer
- perform a calculation using more than one step or type of calculation to produce the correct answer

The aim of this chapter is to present calculations in a simulated real-life situation. Pharmacists presented with checking prescriptions or answering queries from other healthcare professionals may need to retrieve the correct information about a drug, before performing a calculation. For example, in practice an individual drug may be used to treat several different disease states, each disease state often requiring a different dose, dosage form, formulation, etc. Similarly, the dose and dosage regimen may differ depending on the age and or weight of the patient. The ability to retrieve the correct information from information source(s) is an essential skill. In addition, a calculation using retrieved information may involve several steps or the use of more than one concept, e.g. the calculation of a dose based on body weight and the calculation of a percentage solution. Thus, the ability to perform different types of calculations correctly is as important as the ability to retrieve the correct information.

Previously in this book, readers have been given all the information in the question to perform the calculation. This chapter sets out to provide examples where information retrieval is essential before performing the calculation.

In this chapter, profiles of a number of exemplar drugs are provided. Each profile includes details, as appropriate, of dose (by age/weight/route of administration/disease state), formulations available with quantitative details and such information as salts, molecular weights.

Calculations are based only on the exemplar drug profiles provided in the chapter. Each calculation requires the reader initially to retrieve information from the profiles and use this information to perform the calculation. The calculations normally require more than one simple step and/or the performance of more than one type of calculation. Each drug profile is followed by a number of questions that relate to that drug.

Drug A profile

Dose

By mouth for mild infections: adults and children over 8 years, 500 mg every 6 hours or 1 g every 12 hours; neonates 12.5 mg/kg every 6 hours; child 1 month to 2 years 125 mg every 6 hours and 2–8 years 250 mg every 6 hours.

Early syphilis: 500 mg four times daily for 14 days.

By intravenous infusion: adult and child severe infections 50 mg/kg daily by continuous infusion; mild infections (where oral treatment not possible) 25 mg/kg daily.

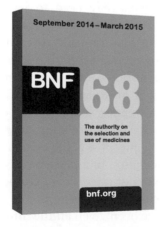

Formulations available:

Tablets	Drug A 250 mg
	Drug A (as stearate) 250 mg
Oral suspension	Drug A (as ethyl succinate) 125 mg/5 mL, 250 mg/5 mL, 500 mg/5 mL
Intravenous infusion powder for reconstitution	Drug A (as lactobionate) 1-g vial

Answer the following questions that relate to drug A.

Q1 A patient who has difficulty swallowing tablets has been diagnosed with early syphilis. What dose and strength of suspension of drug A would you prescribe for this patient to take at home? What total quantity of this suspension would you prescribe for a complete course of treatment? What is the total quantity (in g) of drug A prescribed?

Q2 A neonate (weighing 3.5 kg) with a mild infection requires treatment with drug A. The prescriber decides to use the oral route. What dose and daily dose of drug A should be given to the child? Which strength of suspension should be used and how much of this suspension should be given for each dose?

Q3 A child aged 5 years has a severe infection and requires an intravenous infusion of drug A. What is the total dose of drug A required for 24 hours for this child and what is the dose in mg/hour? Assuming that a vial of drug A is made up to 500 mL, what volume of infusion fluid should be given per hour? What is the concentration (as a percentage) of drug A in the infusion fluid?

Drug B profile

Dose

Anaerobic infections treated for 7 days: by mouth, 800 mg initially then 400 mg every 8 hours and child 7.5 mg/kg every 8 hours; by rectum, 1 g every 8 hours for 3 days, then 1 g every 12 hours; by intravenous infusion over 20 minutes, 500 mg every 8 hours and child 7.5 mg/kg every 8 hours.

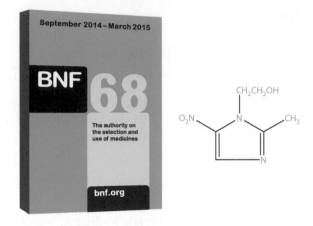

Acute oral infections, by mouth: 200 mg every 8 hours for 5 days; child 1–3 years 50 mg every 8 hours for 5 days; 3–7 years 100 mg every 12 hours; 7–10 years 100 mg every 8 hours.

Formulations available:

Tablets	Drug B 200 mg, 400 mg, 500 mg
Suppositories	Drug B 500 mg and 1 g
Suspension	Drug B 200 mg/5 mL
Intravenous infusion	Drug B 5 mg/mL supplied in 20-mL and 100-mL containers

Answer the following questions that relate to drug B.

Q4 An adult patient with an anaerobic infection requires a course of treatment with drug B. How many tablets of what strength should be supplied for one course?

Q5 A 2-year-old girl has an acute oral infection and requires a course of oral treatment with drug B. She is unable to take tablets but can swallow liquids. What formulation should be supplied? Calculate the amount of formulation to be supplied for each dose, daily dose and total treatment.

Q6 A 10-year-old boy, weighing 30 kg, requires oral treatment with drug B for an anaerobic infection. He cannot swallow tablets and so a liquid formulation is preferred. Calculate the dose and total volume of suspension to be supplied. Calculate your answer to one decimal place.

Q7 An elderly patient with swallowing difficulties requires suppositories to treat an anaerobic infection. Only suppositories containing 500 mg of drug B are available. She requires a dose of 1 g twice daily. Calculate the number of suppositories required for a dose and the total number required for a 7-day course of treatment.

Q8 A child with an anaerobic infection requires treatment by intravenous infusion of drug B. The child is 3 years old and weighs 15 kg. Calculate the dose required. What volume of intravenous infusion will supply this dose?

Drug C profile

Dose

For infections, by mouth: females 500 mg daily in two divided doses, males 600 mg daily in three divided doses; child 3 months to 6 years 360 mg/m^2 daily in four divided doses, 6–12 years 480 mg/m^2 daily in four divided doses.

For patients unable to take drug C by mouth, intravenous infusion 2 mg/kg every 4 hours, child 3 months to 6 years 80 mg/m^2 every 6 hours, 6–12 years 160 mg/m^2.

Formulations available:

Capsules	Drug C 100 mg and 250 mg
Oral solution	Drug C 50 mg/mL
Intravenous infusion	Drug C 10 mg/mL

Answer the following questions that relate to drug C.

Q9 A 1-year-old child requires treatment with drug C by the oral route. The child is unable to swallow capsules but can swallow liquids. What formulation should be provided? Calculate the individual dose, the daily dose and the amount of formulation that should be dispensed for a 14-day supply.

Q10 The above child becomes temporarily unable to take medicines by mouth and is prescribed the equivalent dose by intravenous infusion. What is the dose to be given every 6 hours? What volume of intravenous infusion will contain this dose?

Q11 Calculate the dose of drug C for a woman and the number of capsules of which strength should be prescribed for a course of treatment lasting 21 days.

Q12 Calculate the daily intravenous dose for a man weighing 68 kg. What volume of intravenous infusion of drug C should be administered for each dose?

Drug D profile

Drug D is available as two different salts.
The molecular weights are as follows:

Drug D   749

Drug D salt X   785

Drug D salt Y   860

Dose

Adult 500 mg on the first day, then 250 mg daily for 4 days; child up to 6 months 10 mg/kg once daily for 3 days; body weight 15–35 kg 300 mg once daily for 3 days; body weight 36–45 kg 400 mg once daily for 3 days.

Formulations available:

Tablets   Drug D (as salt Y)   250 mg and 500 mg

Capsules   Drug D (as salt X)   250 mg

Suspension   Drug D (as salt Y)   200 mg in 5 mL

Answer the following questions that relate to drug D.

Q13 Calculate (in grams) the amount of drug D as salt Y that will be required to produce 1 litre of suspension.

Q14 An adult patient is prescribed capsules of drug D at the recommended dose. Calculate the total amount (in grams) of drug D (as salt X) prescribed for the patient.

Q15 A 1-year-old child of normal body weight requires treatment with drug D. Suspension is the formulation of choice. Calculate the amount of suspension required for each dose and the total volume of suspension required for the treatment course. What is the total amount of drug D as salt Y provided for the child?

Drug E profile

Drug E is available as the trihydrate with a molecular weight of 224. This drug becomes classified as a Schedule 2 Controlled Drug when it contains more than the equivalent of 0.5 g of the anhydrous base in 200 mL of a liquid preparation. Below 0.002 g of anhydrous base in 200 mL, it becomes legally classified as a general sales list (GSL) medicine and thus can be freely sold over the counter to customers.

Answer the following questions that relate to drug E.

Q16 A pharmacist prepares a 100 mL of a 0.4% w/v solution of the trihydrate of drug E. Would this solution be classified as a Schedule 2 Controlled Drug?

Q17 A patient is required to take 5 mL four times daily of a 0.1 % w/v solution of drug E (as the anhydrous base) for 14 days. The pharmacist prepares this solution with the trihydrate of drug E. How much of the trihydrate is required to prepare the total volume required by this patient?

Q18 A patient asks if they can buy a 100 mL of a solution containing 500 micrograms of drug E. Calculate if this is legally possible for such a solution. How many milligrams of the trihydrate of drug E will be contained in 500 mL of such a solution?

Drug F profile

Note: 2.2 mg of drug F provides approx. 1 mg of fluoride ion.

Dose

Expressed as fluoride ion (F⁻).

Water content of fluoride ion less than 300 micrograms/L (0.3 ppm): child 6 months–3 years F⁻ 250 micrograms daily, 3–6 years F⁻ 500 micrograms daily, over 6 years F⁻ 1 mg daily.

Water content of fluoride ion between 300 and 700 micrograms/L (0.3–0.7 ppm): child up to 3 years none, 3–6 years F⁻ 250 micrograms daily, over 6 years F⁻ 500 micrograms daily.

Formulations:

Tablets (scored)	1.1 mg and 2.2 mg
Oral drops	550 micrograms/0.15 mL (80 micrograms/drop)
Mouthwash	0.55% and 2%
Toothpaste	0.62% and 1.1%

Answer the following questions that relate to drug F.

Q19 A 7-year-old child lives in an area in which the tap water contains F⁻ 500 micrograms/L. What strength of tablet should be prescribed at the recommended dosage and how many would provide treatment for 14 days. How much fluoride ion would be provided by the total treatment (give your answer in milligrams)?

Q20 A sibling, aged 4 years, of the above child requires drug F. The parent would like to use the same strength tablets as those prescribed to the older child. What is the dose for the younger child and how could this be given using the same strength tablets?

Q21 A child is prescribed 360 micrograms of fluoride ion per day. How many drops of the oral drops should be given per day to provide this dose? What is the percentage concentration of fluoride ion in the oral drops?

Q22 A healthcare professional asks you how much fluoride ion is contained in a 10 mL quantity of 0.55% mouthwash and a similar quantity of 2% mouthwash. What is your answer?

Q23 A healthcare professional tells you that the local tap water contains 4 ppm of fluoride ion. They want to know if toothpaste containing drug F contains more or less than this. Calculate the fluoride concentration in parts per million of both strengths of toothpaste.

A1   Daily dose of suspension is 5 mL four times a day of 500 mg/5 mL

Total volume of suspension is 280 mL

Total quantity of drug A is 28 g

A2   Dose = 43.75 mg

Daily dose = 87.5 mg

Dose of drug A is 1.75 mL of a suspension containing 125 mg/ 5 mL

A3   900 mg in 24 hours

18.75 mL of infusion fluid will supply 37.5 mg of drug A and should be given per hour

Concentration of infusion fluid is 0.2%

A4   22 tablets of 400 mg

A5   1.25 mL of suspension will provide the dose of 50 mg

3.75 mL of suspension will provide the daily dose

18.75 mL is the total amount for the course of treatment

A6   Dose is 5.62 mL of suspension Total volume is 117.6 mL

A7   Two 500-mg suppositories for each dose

Total number of 500-mg suppositories required is 28

A8   Dose is 112.5 mg

Volume of intravenous infusion is 22.5 mL

A9   Oral solution

Daily dose is $0.49 \times 360 =$ 176 mg

Each individual dose is 44 mg approx. 4.5 mL of suspension

Total for 14 days is 238 mL

A10   Dose is 37 mg

3.7 mL will contain the correct dose

A11   Dose is 500 mg daily in two divided doses, so 250 mg per dose

Provide 42 capsules each containing 250 mg

A12   Daily dose is 816 mg based on six doses in 24 hours

Each dose is provided by 13.6 mL of intravenous infusion

A13   45.93 g of salt Y

A14   1.572 g of salt X of drug D

A15   Each dose is 2.25 mL of suspension

Total volume of suspension is 6.75 mL

Total amount of drug D as salt Y is 310 mg

A16   Yes. Solution contains 0.3% w/v of the anhydrous base which is above the concentration for a Schedule 2 Controlled Drug

A17   Total amount of trihydrate required is 0.369 g

A18 0.0005 g in 100 mL is below 0.002 g in 200 mL (0.001 g/100 mL) and can be sold

500 mL of solution will contain 3.3 mg of the trihydrate

A19 14 tablets of 1.1 mg
Total fluoride ion is 7 mg

A20 Dose is 500 micrograms, so half a 1.1-mg tablet

A21 10 drops/day
0.14% w/v of fluoride ion

A22 10 mL of 2% mouthwash contains 90.9 mg of fluoride ion

10 mL of 0.55% mouthwash contains 25 mg fluoride ion

A23 0.62% toothpaste contains 2810 ppm

1.1% toothpaste contains 5000 ppm

Appendix 1

Metric prefixes

exa	E	10^{18}
peta	P	10^{15}
tera	T	10^{12}
giga	G	10^{9}
mega	M	10^{6}
kilo	k	10^{3}
hecto	h	10^{2}
deca	da	10
deci	d	10^{-1}
centi	c	10^{-2}
milli	m	10^{-3}
micro	mc or μ*	10^{-6}
nano	n*	10^{-9}
pico	p	10^{-12}
femto	f	10^{-15}
atto	a	10^{-18}

*micrograms and nanograms should not be abbreviated in prescription writing

Appendix 2

Conversion factors

Mass

1 ounce (oz) = 28.35 grams (g)

1 pound (lb) = 16 ounces = 0.4536 kilogram (kg)

1 stone (st) = 14 pounds = 6.35 kg

1 kilogram = 2.205 lb

Length

1 inch (in) = 25.4 millimetres (mm)

1 foot (ft) = 12 inches = 304.8 millimetres (mm)

1 yard = 3 feet = 914.8 millimetres (mm)

1 mile = 1760 yards = 1.609 kilometres (km)

1 metre (m) = 3.282 feet

Volume

1 pint = 20 fluid ounces (fl. oz.) = 568 millilitres (mL)

1 gallon = 8 pints = 4.546 litres (L)

1 litre (L) = 1.76 pints

Other units

1 kilocalorie (kcal) = 4186.8 joules (J)

1 millimetre of mercury (mmHg) = 133.3 pascals (Pa)

Appendix 3

Multiplication and division

The following methods for multiplication and division of integers and fractions are included for reference.

Multiplication

Long multiplication

Example A3.1

Multiply 3576 by 34

Write the numbers below each other, with right side aligned:

$$3576$$
$$34$$

$3576 \times 4 = 14\,304$ and write below line

$3576 \times 30 = 107\,280$ and write below previous number

Add the numbers below the line together to give the answer

14 304	
107 280	
121 584	

Therefore, $3576 \times 34 = 121\,584$.

Example A3.2

Multiply 2187 by 356

Write the numbers below each other with right side aligned:

$$2187$$
$$356$$

(continued)

$2187 \times 6 = 13\,122$ and write below line	$13\,122$
$2187 \times 50 = 109\,350$ and write below previous number	$109\,350$
$2187 \times 300 = 656\,100$ and write below previous number	$656\,100$
Add the numbers below the line together to give the answer	$778\,572$

Therefore, $2187 \times 356 = 778\,572$.

Multiplication of a fraction by another fraction

Example A3.3

Multiply $\dfrac{2}{5}$ by $\dfrac{3}{4}$

Multiply the numerators $2 \times 3 = 6$

Multiply the denominators $5 \times 4 = 20$

Place the product of the numerators over the product of the denominators: $\dfrac{6}{20}$

Simplify by dividing the numerator and denominator by the same number (in this case 2) $= \dfrac{3}{10}$

Therefore: $\dfrac{2}{5} \times \dfrac{3}{4} = \dfrac{3}{10}$

Example A3.4

Multiply $\dfrac{2}{35}$ by $\dfrac{3}{24}$

Multiply the numerators $2 \times 3 = 6$

Multiply the denominators $35 \times 24 = 840$

→

Place the product of the numerators over the product of the denominators: $\dfrac{6}{840}$

By dividing the numerator and denominator by 6 we simplify the fraction to $\dfrac{1}{140}$

Therefore: $\dfrac{2}{35} \times \dfrac{3}{24} = \dfrac{1}{140}$

An alternative way to do the above multiplication is to 'cancel' before doing the multiplication.

$\dfrac{2}{35} \times \dfrac{3}{24}$ can be expressed as $\dfrac{2 \times 3}{35 \times 24}$

Again, as long as we do the same to both the numerator and the denominator the fraction remains in the same ratio and is therefore equal. This is also true if we divide one factor in the numerator and one factor in the denominator by the same figure.

So we could divide the 2 and the 24 by 2 giving 1 and 12.

We could then divide the 3 and the 12 by 3 to get 1 and 4.

So the sum becomes $\dfrac{1 \times 1}{35 \times 4} = \dfrac{1}{140}$

Multiplication of a decimal

Example A3.5

Multiply 5.2 by 6.95

First consider the numbers without the decimal points and multiply:

$52 \times 695 = 36140$

The sum of the number of figures after the decimal point for both factors $= 3$.

Count three figures from the right hand side of the product towards the left and put the point to the left of this figure $= 36.140$.

Example A3.6

Multiply 5.78 by 9.75

Again ignore the decimal points and multiply using the method described previously:

$578 \times 975 = 563\,550$

The sum of the number of figures after the decimal place in the two factors $= 4$.

Count four figures from the right hand side of the product towards the left and put the point to the left of this figure $= 56.3550$.

Division

Long division

A simple mnemonic to remember the stages involved in long division is DMSB which stands for divide, multiply, subtract and bring down. (Remember it by dad, mum, sister, brother or does Macdonald's sell burgers?)
The process is as follows:

Example A3.7

Divide 6642 by 18 $18\overline{)6642}$

Divide the 18 into the figure starting at the digit on the left, i.e. 6. We start by dividing 18 into 6 goes 0 times or will not go. So we then consider the next digit, again a 6 and ask the question how many times does 18 go into 66. Answer 3.

Multiply 3×18

Subtract the 54 from 66

$$
\begin{array}{r}
3 \\
18\overline{)6642} \\
54 \\
\hline
12 \rightarrow
\end{array}
$$

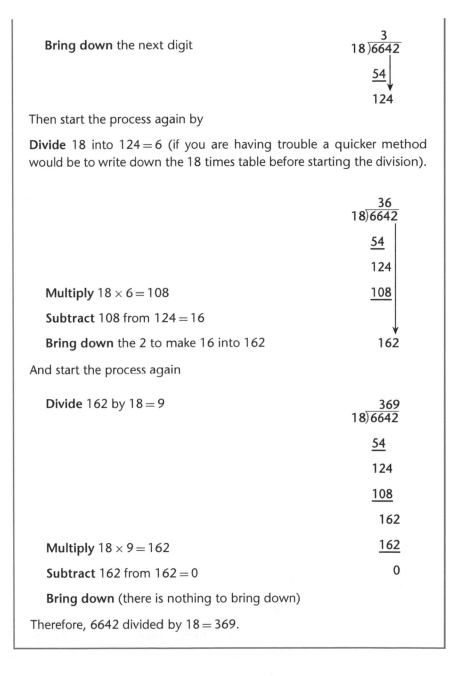

Bring down the next digit

$$18\overline{)6642}^{\,3}$$

Then start the process again by

Divide 18 into 124 = 6 (if you are having trouble a quicker method would be to write down the 18 times table before starting the division).

Multiply 18 × 6 = 108

Subtract 108 from 124 = 16

Bring down the 2 to make 16 into 162

And start the process again

Divide 162 by 18 = 9

Multiply 18 × 9 = 162

Subtract 162 from 162 = 0

Bring down (there is nothing to bring down)

Therefore, 6642 divided by 18 = 369.

If there was remainder at the end of the units then you would bring down a zero as the next number and place a decimal point in the answer.

Example A3.8

19 divided by 16 $16\overline{)19}$

16 into 1 goes 0, bring down the next number.

$$\begin{array}{r} 1 \\ 16\overline{)19} \end{array}$$

  Divide 16 into 19 goes 1

  Multiply $1 \times 16 = 16$ 16

  Subtract $19 - 16 = 3$ 3

So the answer is 1 remainder 3

This could also be expressed as $1\dfrac{3}{16}$

We can consider 19 being the same as 19.00000 so we can continue to **divide** the number but we also put a decimal point in the answer 1.

$$\begin{array}{r} 1. \\ 16\overline{)19.0} \end{array}$$

  Multiply $1 \times 16 = 16$ 16

  Subtract $19 - 16 = 3$

  Bring down the zero and put decimal point in answer   30

Then start the process again:

  Divide 30 by $16 = 1$

$$\begin{array}{r} 1.1 \\ 16\overline{)19.00} \end{array}$$

                                                                     16

                                                                     30

  Multiply $16 \times 1 = 16$ 16

  Subtract $30 - 16 = 14$

  Bring down the next 0 to make 14   140

And again we repeat the process until there is no remainder or enough decimal places have been reached.

Therefore, 19 divided by $16 = 1.1875$.

Dividing a fraction by another fraction

To do this we can invert the denominator fraction and multiply the fractions as before.

Example A3.9

Divide $\dfrac{1}{24}$ by $\dfrac{3}{16} = \dfrac{1}{24} \times \dfrac{16}{3}$

$\dfrac{1 \times 16}{24 \times 3} = \dfrac{16}{72}$

Simplify by dividing the numerator and denominator by $8 = \dfrac{2}{9}$.

Therefore: $\dfrac{1}{24}$ divided by $\dfrac{3}{16} = \dfrac{2}{9}$.

Dividing decimals by decimals

Example A3.10

49.68 divided by 3.6

Change the denominator fraction to an integer 36 (by multiplying by 10).

Multiply the numerator fraction by the same number $49.68 \times 10 = 496.8$.

Conduct a long division:

Divide 49 by $36 = 1$

Multiply $36 \times 1 = 36$

Subtract $49 - 36 = 13$

Bring down the 6

$$
\begin{array}{r}
1 \\
36\overline{)496.8} \\
36 \\
\hline
136
\end{array}
$$

(continued)

Divide 136 by 36 = 3

$$
\begin{array}{r}
13. \\
36\overline{)496.8} \\
\underline{36} \\
136 \\
\end{array}
$$

Multiply 36 × 3 = 108

$$\underline{108}$$

Subtract 136 − 108 = 28

Bring down the 8 and put a decimal point in the answer

288

Divide 288 by 36 = 8

$$
\begin{array}{r}
13.8 \\
36\overline{)496.8} \\
\underline{36} \\
136 \\
\underline{108} \\
288 \\
\end{array}
$$

Multiply 36 × 8 = 288

$$\underline{288}$$

Subtract 288 − 288 = 0

0

Therefore, 49.68 divided by 3.6 = 13.8.

Appendix 4

Atomic weights of the elements ($^{12}C = 12$)

Atomic number	Name	Symbol	Atomic weight
89	Actinium	Ac	*
13	Aluminium	Al	26.981 538
95	Americium	Am	*
51	Antimony	Sb	121.760
18	Argon	Ar	39.948
33	Arsenic	As	74.921 60
85	Astatine	At	*
56	Barium	Ba	137.327
97	Berkelium	Bk	*
4	Beryllium	Be	9.012 182
83	Bismuth	Bi	208.980 38
107	Bohrium	Bh	*
5	Boron	B	10.811
35	Bromine	Br	79.904
48	Cadmium	Cd	112.411
55	Caesium	Cs	132.905 45
20	Calcium	Ca	40.078
98	Californium	Cf	*
6	Carbon	C	12.0107

continued overleaf

Atomic number	Name	Symbol	Atomic weight
58	Cerium	Ce	140.116
17	Chlorine	Cl	35.4527
24	Chromium	Cr	51.9961
27	Cobalt	Co	58.933 200
29	Copper	Cu	63.546
96	Curium	Cm	*
105	Dubnium	Db	*
66	Dysprosium	Dy	162.50
99	Einsteinium	Es	*
68	Erbium	Er	167.26
63	Europium	Eu	151.964
100	Fermium	Fm	*
9	Fluorine	F	18.998 403 2
87	Francium	Fr	*
64	Gadolinium	Gd	157.25
31	Gallium	Ga	69.723
32	Germanium	Ge	72.61
79	Gold	Au	196.966 55
72	Hafnium	Hf	178.49
108	Hassium	Hs	*
2	Helium	He	4.002 602
67	Holmium	Ho	164.930 32
1	Hydrogen	H	1.007 94
49	Indium	In	114.818
53	Iodine	I	126.904 47
77	Iridium	Ir	192.217

$\longrightarrow$

26	Iron	Fe	55.845
36	Krypton	Kr	83.80
57	Lanthanum	La	138.9055
103	Lawrencium	Lr	*
82	Lead	Pb	207.2
3	‡Lithium	Li	6.941
71	Lutetium	Lu	174.967
12	Magnesium	Mg	24.3050
25	Manganese	Mn	54.938 049
109	Meitnerium	Mt	*
101	Mendelevium	Md	*
80	Mercury	Hg	200.59
42	Molybdenum	Mo	95.94
60	Neodymium	Nd	144.24
10	Neon	Ne	20.1797
93	Neptunium	Np	*
28	Nickel	Ni	58.6934
41	Niobium	Nb	92.906 38
7	Nitrogen	N	14.006 74
102	Nobelium	No	*
76	Osmium	Os	190.23
8	Oxygen	O	15.9994
46	Palladium	Pd	106.42
15	Phosphorus	P	30.973 761
78	Platinum	Pt	195.078
94	Plutonium	Pu	*
84	Polonium	Po	*

continued overleaf

Atomic number	Name	Symbol	Atomic weight
19	Potassium	K	39.0983
59	Praseodymium	Pr	140.907 65
61	Promethium	Pm	*
91	†Protactinium	Pa	231.035 88
88	Radium	Ra	*
86	Radon	Rn	*
75	Rhenium	Re	186.207
45	Rhodium	Rh	102.905 50
37	Rubidium	Rb	85.4678
44	Ruthenium	Ru	101.07
104	Rutherfordium	Rf	*
62	Samarium	Sm	150.36
21	Scandium	Sc	44.955 910
106	Seaborgium	Sg	*
34	Selenium	Se	78.96
14	Silicon	Si	28.0855
47	Silver	Ag	107.8682
11	Sodium	Na	22.989 770
38	Strontium	Sr	87.62
16	Sulfur	S	32.066
73	Tantalum	Ta	180.9479
43	Technetium	Tc	*
52	Tellurium	Te	127.60
65	Terbium	Tb	158.925 34
81	Thallium	Tl	204.3833
90	†Thorium	Th	232.0381

$\longrightarrow$

69	Thulium	Tm	168.934 21
50	Tin	Sn	118.710
22	Titanium	Ti	47.867
74	Tungsten	W	183.84
110	Ununnilium	Uun	*
111	Unununium	Uuu	*
92	†Uranium	U	238.0289
23	Vanadium	V	50.9415
54	Xenon	Xe	131.29
70	Ytterbium	Yb	173.04
39	Yttrium	Y	88.905 85
30	Zinc	Zn	65.39
40	Zirconium	Zr	91.224

*Elements marked * have no stable nuclides and IUPAC states 'there is no general agreement on which of the isotopes of the radioactive elements is, or is likely to be judged "important" and various criteria such as "longest half-life", "production in quantity", "used commercially", etc., have been applied in the Commission's choice.' However, atomic weights are given for radioactive elements marked † as they do have a characteristic terrestrial isotopic composition. Commercially available lithium (‡) materials have atomic weights ranging from 6.94 to 6.99; if a more accurate value is required, it must be determined for the specific material.

Appendix 5

Body surface area in children

Body weight under 40 kg

Body weight (kg)	Surface area (m²)
1	0.10
1.5	0.13
2	0.16
2.5	0.19
3	0.21
3.5	0.24
4	0.26
4.5	0.28
5	0.30
5.5	0.32
6	0.34
6.5	0.36
7	0.38
7.5	0.40
8	0.42
8.5	0.44
9	0.46

continued overleaf

Body weight (kg)	Surface area (m²)
9.5	0.47
10	0.49
11	0.53
12	0.56
13	0.59
14	0.62
15	0.65
16	0.68
17	0.71
18	0.74
19	0.77
20	0.79
21	0.82
22	0.85
23	0.87
24	0.90
25	0.92
26	0.95
27	0.97
28	1.0
29	1.0
30	1.1
31	1.1
32	1.1
33	1.1
34	1.1

$\longrightarrow$

Body weight (kg)	Surface area (m²)
35	1.2
36	1.2
37	1.2
38	1.2
39	1.3
40	1.3

Values are calculated using the Boyd equation
Note: Height is not required to estimate body surface area using these tables

Body weight over 40 kg

Body weight (kg)	Surface area (m²)
41	1.3
42	1.3
43	1.3
44	1.4
45	1.4
46	1.4
47	1.4
48	1.4
49	1.5
50	1.5
51	1.5
52	1.5
53	1.5
54	1.6
55	1.6

continued overleaf

Body weight (kg)	Surface area (m²)
56	1.6
57	1.6
58	1.6
59	1.7
60	1.7
61	1.7
62	1.7
63	1.7
64	1.7
65	1.8
66	1.8
67	1.8
68	1.8
69	1.8
70	1.9
71	1.9
72	1.9
73	1.9
74	1.9
75	1.9
76	2.0
77	2.0
78	2.0
79	2.0
80	2.0
81	2.0

$\longrightarrow$

82	2.1
83	2.1
84	2.1
85	2.1
86	2.1
87	2.1
88	2.2
89	2.2
90	2.2

Values are calculated using the Boyd equation

Note: Height is not required to estimate body surface area using these tables

Adapted by permission from Macmillan Publishers Ltd: Sharkey I et al, *British Journal of Cancer* 2001; 85 (1): 23–28, © 2001. Reproduced by permission from *BNF for Children*; Copyright © BMJ Group, RPS Publishing, RCPCH Publication Ltd 2009.

Bibliography

British Pharmacopoeia, current edition. London: Stationery Office (updated annually).

British National Formulary. [current edition] ed. London: British Medical Association and Royal Pharmaceutical Society of Great Britain.

Martindale: The complete drug reference, 38th edn (Brayfield A, ed.). London: Pharmaceutical Press, 2014.

Medicines, Ethics and Practice, London: Pharmaceutical Press (published annually in July).

The Pharmaceutical Codex: Principles and practice of pharmaceutics, 12th edn (Lund W, ed.) London: Pharmaceutical Press, 1994.

Index